The McDougall Quick & Easy Cookbook

Over 300 Delicious Low-Fat Recipes You Can Prepare in Fifteen Minutes or Less

The McDougall Quick & Easy Cookbook

John A. McDougall, M.D., and Mary McDougall

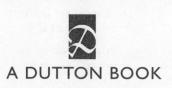
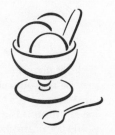

A DUTTON BOOK

DUTTON
Published by the Penguin Group
Penguin Books USA Inc., 375 Hudson Street, New York, New York 10014, U.S.A.
Penguin Books Ltd, 27 Wrights Lane, London W8 5TZ, England
Penguin Books Australia Ltd, Ringwood, Victoria, Australia
Penguin Books Canada Ltd, 10 Alcorn Avenue, Toronto, Ontario, Canada M4V 3B2
Penguin Books (N.Z.) Ltd, 182–190 Wairau Road, Auckland 10, New Zealand

Penguin Books Ltd, Registered Offices: Harmondsworth, Middlesex, England

First published by Dutton, an imprint of Dutton Signet,
a division of Penguin Books USA Inc.
Distributed in Canada by McClelland & Stewart Inc.

First Printing, August, 1997
10 9 8 7 6 5 4 3 2 1

 REGISTERED TRADEMARK—MARCA REGISTRADA

LIBRARY OF CONGRESS CATALOGING-IN-PUBLICATION DATA:
McDougall, John A.
The McDougall quick and easy cookbook : over 300 delicious recipes you can
prepare in fifteen minutes or less / John A. McDougall and Mary McDougall.
p.   cm.
Includes index.
ISBN 0-525-94208-4
1. Low-fat diet—Recipes.   I. McDougall, Mary A. (Mary Ann)   II. Title.
RM237.7M417   1997
641.5'638—dc21   97-3453
CIP

Printed in the United States of America
Set in Garamond Book
Artwork by Lisa Kahn

To the modern-day homemaker/breadwinner/parent/husband or wife/community project member/PTA volunteer who deserves, after a hard day's work, great-tasting, effortless meals.

Acknowledgments

∙∙

Our gratitude and thanks to:

Lisa Kahn of Mona Lisa Designs for providing the artwork for our book. Silver Tree, a dedicated employee of The McDougall Wellness Center, for researching the product list. A very special thanks to all of you who sent us your suggestions and recipes; a list of the contributors is found on page 309. (Our apologies to anyone we overlooked.) Dr. McDougall's Right Foods, the mission-oriented company that has made great health effortless. The McDougall Program at St. Helena Hospital in the Napa Valley, a live-in experience that assures success with the McDougall Program (our professional staff locks you up for twelve days of summer camp). The employees of The McDougall Wellness Center, who make you feel like the most important person in the world when you call for help.

If you have any questions, or ideas you would like to share, please write or call.

The McDougall
  Wellness Center
PO Box 14039
Santa Rosa, CA 95403

Telephone: (707) 576-1654
Book orders: (800) 570-1654
FAX: (707) 576-3313
E-mail: drmcdougall@drmcdougall.com
On the web: http://www.drmcdougall.com

Dr. McDougall's Right Foods
101 Utah Avenue
San Francisco, CA 94080

Telephone: (415) 635-6000
FAX: (415) 635-6010
Food orders: (800) 367-3844
E-mail: drmcdougall@right-foods.com
On the web: http://www.right-foods.com

The McDougall Program/
   St. Helena Hospital
650 Sanitarium Drive
Deer Park, CA 94576

Telephone: (707) 963-6365
Reservations: (800) 358-9195

Contents

Introduction

*Y*ou will no longer have to make a choice between good health and your busy life. All of the recipes in *The McDougall Quick and Easy Cookbook* require 15 minutes or less to prepare and taste better than meals that take hours in the kitchen (cooking times are often longer than 15 minutes). Carefully selected combinations of starches, vegetables, fruits, and spices, time-saving steps and the use of already cooked healthy ingredients are the secrets to the success of these recipes. When Mary read on the radio show the recipe for Speedy International Stew, which contains only three ingredients, she received dozens of comments, all of which expressed the same sentiment, "I never realized such a simple combination of ingredients could taste so great." After just one terrific taste experience you'll dig deeper into the book and discover how delicious easy meals can be.

The book is designed for quick learning as well as fast meals. Scattered throughout the recipes you will find snapshots of essential information on nutrition, medicine, and food. The *recipe section* gives you helpful hints for preparing and serving dishes. Quick tips are provided to speed up easy meals. An up-to-date *canned and pack- aged products list* appears at the end of the book. Read the ingredient labels carefully, because some products may contain ingredients you should avoid for your health.

Diet is powerful medicine, and you need to be prepared for the changes that will take place when you improve the quality of your body's food supply. If like most Americans, you are relatively healthy—just a little fat, constipated, headachy, and arthritic—then you can start the program today without fear of serious side effects. You should expect to see immediate improvements as you start pumping the right fuel into your engine.

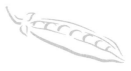

However, if you are seriously ill, you should change your diet only under the supervision of a qualified doctor. You may have special dietary requirements, such as a very low protein and potassium diet for kidney failure. This warning is also important if you are on medication, especially heart, blood pressure, or diabetes medications. You must have a physician's help to adjust your medication—usually to lower or eliminate it—when you change your diet. Diabetes medication can dangerously lower the blood sugar if it is not reduced or stopped when the McDougall diet causes the body's own insulin to work more efficiently. In most cases when you and your doctor are making adjustments, it is better to err on the side of reducing medication sooner, rather than later.

The McDougall Program is ideal nutrition, as well as powerful medicine. One addition you should make if you are following the diet strictly for more than 3 years, or you are pregnant or nursing a baby, is to add a non-animal source of B12 to your diet (5 micrograms daily from a quality vitamin supplement).

The McDougall Quick and Easy Cookbook is a practical resource to help you achieve permanent control over your health and appearance. However, if you are starting the McDougall Program for serious medical problems you should refer to the other McDougall books listed below, which will provide you with essential information.

Recommended McDougall Books:

The McDougall Program—Twelve Days to Dynamic Health
The McDougall Program for a Healthy Heart
The McDougall Program for Maximum Weight Loss
The New McDougall Cookbook
McDougall's Medicine—A Challenging Second Opinion
The McDougall Plan
The McDougall Health-Supporting Cookbooks—Volumes I and II

THE MCDOUGALL STORY

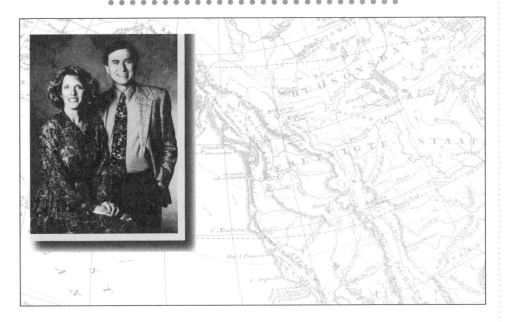

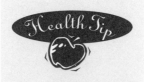

*T*he McDougall Program began where our lives began, in Michigan. I was raised in Grand Rapids and John in the Detroit area. We met while working at Blodgett Hospital in Grand Rapids. After our marriage in 1972 we left for Hawaii, where John did his internship at Queen's Medical Center in Honolulu. The next year we moved to the Big Island of Hawaii.

John worked as a doctor on a sugar plantation, where he discovered the importance of nutrition while taking care of first through fourth-generation Filipinos, Japanese, and Chinese. His older patients, who lived on rice and vegetables, were thin and free of common chronic diseases; however, their children and grandchildren, who began eating a "well-balanced" diet with meat and dairy products, became fat and sick. Obviously the problem wasn't genetics: The change in diet caused the change in their health.

We moved back to Oahu, where John resumed his training and became a board-certified internist. In 1987 we moved to California to run the twelve-day live-in McDougall Program at St. Helena Hospital in the Napa Valley.

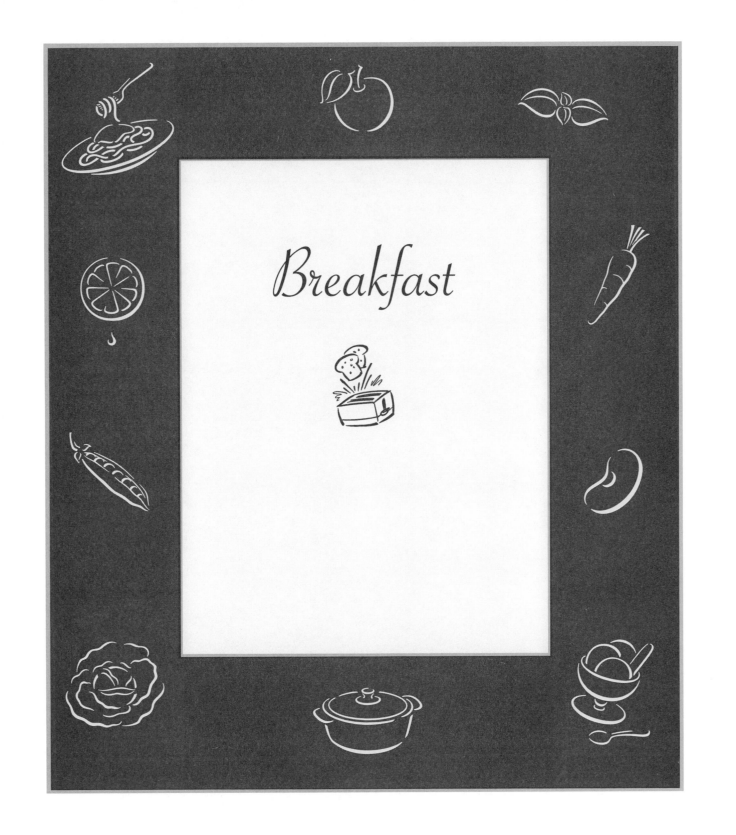

Breakfast

Almost Instant Breakfast

½ cup quick-cooking oatmeal
¼ cup applesauce
1 tablespoon raisins

dash of cinnamon
¾ cup boiling water

Servings: 1
Preparation Time:
5 minutes
Cooking Time:
5 minutes

Combine the oatmeal, applesauce, raisins, and cinnamon in a small covered bowl. Set aside overnight. In the morning, add the boiling water, stir, let rest for 5 minutes, and then eat.

Recipe Hint: Add some sliced bananas when you add the boiling water. This may also be made in the morning, without the overnight rest time, but for some reason it seems quicker when you assemble the ingredients the night before.

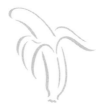

Sweet Breakfast Rice

1 cup cooked brown rice
3 dates

⅓ cup water
¾ whole banana

Servings: 1
Preparation Time:
5 minutes
(need cooked rice)
Cooking Time:
1 minute

Heat the rice in a microwave until warm, about 1 minute. Stir and set aside. Place the dates and water in a blender jar and process briefly. Add the banana and process until smooth. Pour over the warmed rice.

Recipe Hint: Use different dried fruits or frozen fresh fruits. Add vanilla or cinnamon.

Apple Cinnamon Oatmeal

Servings: 2
Preparation Time:
8 minutes
Cooking Time:
5 minutes

1 apple, cored and diced
⅔ cup apple juice
⅔ cup water

¼ teaspoon cinnamon
⅔ cup quick-cooking oatmeal

Combine the apple, juice, water, and cinnamon in a saucepan. Bring to a boil. Stir in the oatmeal and cook for 2 minutes. Remove from heat, cover, and let rest for 1 to 2 minutes before serving.

Crock Pot Rise and Shine

Servings: 4 to 6
Preparation Time:
2 minutes
Cooking Time:
8 to 10 hours

1 cup Stone-Buhr Hot Apple
Granola

5 cups water

Place the granola and water in a Crock Pot. Cover and cook on low heat for 8 to 10 hours.

Recipe Hint: *This cereal has so much flavor built in from the raisins, apples, and cinnamon that your whole family will wake up to these delicious smells in the morning. Variations are easy to make using the same amounts of cereal and water—just use different grains: cracked wheat, oat flakes, barley flakes, whole oats, barley, wheat berries, or brown rice. Add raisins, bits of dried apples, and a dash of cinnamon, nutmeg, and/or mace for extra flavor.*

Breakfast Couscous

¾ cup water
¼ cup orange juice
½ cup couscous
¼ cup raisins

½ cup sliced banana
2 tablespoons frozen apple juice
  concentrate
¼ teaspoon cinnamon

Servings: 2
Preparation Time:
5 minutes
Cooking Time:
5 minutes

Combine all ingredients in a microwave-safe bowl. Cover. Microwave on high for 4 minutes. Remove and let rest for 1 minute. Serve hot.

To prepare on the stovetop, place all ingredients in a saucepan. Bring to a boil, cover, and cook for 5 minutes. Let rest for 3 minutes. Serve hot.

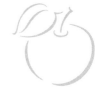

Oatmeal Masa Porridge

⅓ cup quick-cooking oatmeal
¼ cup instant corn masa mix

1¼ cups water

Servings: 1
Preparation Time:
3 minutes
Cooking Time:
4 minutes

Mix the dry ingredients together in a microwave-safe bowl. Slowly stir in the water. Microwave on high for 2 minutes. Stir. Microwave an additional 2 minutes.

To prepare on the stovetop, place all ingredients in a saucepan and mix well. Bring to a boil, stirring frequently. Cook, stirring occasionally, for 5 minutes.

Recipe Hint: Try Maseca brand instant corn masa mix by Azteca Milling Company. The masa mix may be replaced with brown rice flour, whole wheat flour, or cornmeal. To boost the flavor of this porridge, add ½ teaspoon cinnamon to the dry ingredients and 1 mashed banana after the water has been stirred in.

SURGEON GENERAL'S REPORT

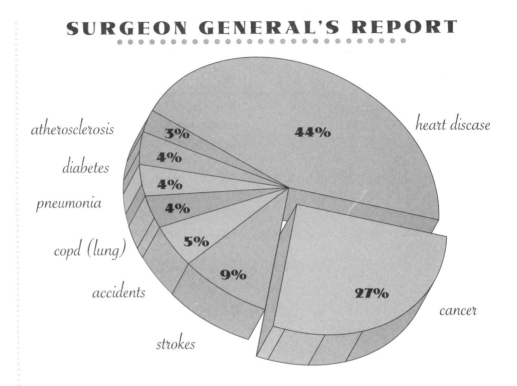

atherosclerosis — 3%
diabetes — 4%
pneumonia — 4%
copd (lung) — 4%
accidents — 5%
strokes — 9%
heart disease — 44%
cancer — 27%

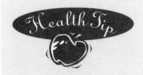

Grandma said, "You are what you eat." And the consensus of scientific opinion agrees: The way we eat and live determines our present and future health.

*A*ccording to the Surgeon General, the leading cause of death and disability for Americans is our rich diet. Several hundred of the country's top scientists conducted a thorough review of the scientific literature. Their findings, contained in the Surgeon General's Report on Nutrition and Health, revealed that five of the ten leading causes of death—heart disease, cancer, stroke, diabetes, and atherosclerosis—are due to the foods we eat and therefore potentially preventable. When the impact of alcohol is considered, four more causes of death are added to the top-ten list: accidents, suicides, homicides, and cirrhosis of the liver.

People who believe that disease is caused by events beyond our control—heredity, bad luck, the wrath of God—are helpless victims. By acting on the Surgeon General's message, we control our future and reduce our risk of premature death from nine of the ten leading causes. Of the 2.1 million people who died in 1987, 1.5 million died as a consequence of what they ate or drank.

Jack's Breakfast Sandwich

1 large baking potato
4 slices whole wheat bread

2 tablespoons ketchup

Servings: 2
Preparation Time:
5 minutes
Cooking Time:
13 minutes

Scrub the potato and prick all over with a fork. Microwave on high for 3 minutes. Remove the potato and thickly slice lengthwise. Place on a nonstick griddle and brown on both sides for about 10 minutes.

Spread the bread with ketchup, place the potato slices on the bread, and serve at once.

Recipe Hint: *If you prefer, toast the bread before spreading it with ketchup. This is a fast and easy breakfast that can be eaten on the run.*

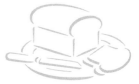

Applesauce Pancakes

1 cup unbleached white flour
½ cup whole wheat flour
1½ teaspoons baking powder
1 cup rice milk

¾ cup applesauce
1 teaspoon vanilla extract
1 teaspoon egg replacer mixed
   with 2 tablespoons water

Servings: makes
12 pancakes
Preparation Time:
10 minutes
Cooking Time:
20 minutes

Mix the dry ingredients together (except the egg replacer) in a bowl. Mix the wet ingredients together. In a separate bowl, beat the egg replacer and water until very frothy. Add to the wet ingredients. Combine the wet and dry ingredients and beat until well blended. Pour the batter onto a hot nonstick griddle. When bubbles form on top of the pancakes and the edges are beginning to dry out, turn to bake the other side. To serve, spread a little applesauce over them and sprinkle with cinnamon.

Recipe Hint: *Use a wooden spoon to mix wet and dry ingredients only until the dry ingredients are moistened. Overmixing will make the finished product dense and hard.*

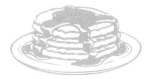

Banana French Toast

Servings: 6
Preparation Time:
5 minutes
Cooking Time:
8 minutes

**1 banana, broken into large
  pieces**
½ cup soy milk

1 teaspoon vanilla extract
¾ teaspoon cinnamon
6 slices bread

Place the banana, soy milk, vanilla, and cinnamon in a blender jar. Process until smooth. Transfer to a shallow bowl. Dip the bread in the batter and cook on a nonstick griddle for about 2 minutes on each side.

> **Recipe Hint:** *Make sure the griddle is hot before adding the bread to it. For the best results, use an Italian-style bread rather than a dense bread to allow the batter to soak into the bread slightly.*

Lite French Toast

Servings: 6
Preparation Time:
5 minutes
Cooking Time:
8 minutes

1 cup rice milk
¼ teaspoon vanilla extract
¼ teaspoon cinnamon

pinch of nutmeg
6 slices whole wheat bread

Combine all ingredients, except the bread, in a bowl, mixing well. Dip the bread slices into the mixture, coating both sides well.

Cook on a nonstick griddle for about 2 minutes on each side, turning once until browned on both sides. Serve with pure maple syrup, applesauce, or fruit jam.

Nutty French Toast

¼ cup raw cashews
1 cup water
2 tablespoons chopped dates
½ teaspoon vanilla extract

¼ teaspoon cinnamon
dash of turmeric
6 slices whole wheat bread

Servings: 6
Preparation Time:
5 minutes
Cooking Time:
8 minutes

Place the cashews in a blender jar with ½ cup of the water. Process until fairly smooth, then add the remaining ½ cup water and the dates, vanilla, cinnamon, and turmeric. Process until very smooth. Pour into a bowl. Dip the bread slices into the mixture, coating both sides well. Cook on a nonstick griddle for about 2 minutes on each side, turning once until browned on both sides.

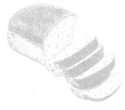

Recipe Hint: *Make sure the griddle is hot before you cook the first slice. Test by sprinkling a few drops of water on it—they bounce when the griddle is ready. Serve French toast with pure maple syrup, applesauce, or fruit jam.*

Veggie Benedicts

2 nonfat English muffins, split in
  half
4 thick slices tomato

1 small avocado, peeled and sliced
1 cup Hollandaise Sauce
  (page 234)

Servings: 4
Preparation Time:
5 minutes
(need prepared
Hollandaise Sauce)
Cooking Time:
2 to 3 minutes

Place the muffins in a toaster or toaster oven and toast until lightly browned.

Place a tomato slice on each muffin and then the avocado slices. Pour ¼ of the sauce over each muffin and serve at once.

Recipe Hint: *This is a treat we enjoy for special occasions. Sometimes we use steamed broccoli florets in place of the avocado. Nonfat crumpets may be used in place of the English muffins.*

Scrambled Tofu

Servings: 4
Preparation Time:
10 minutes
Cooking Time:
10 minutes

½ cup water
1 onion, chopped
½ cup chopped green bell pepper
½ cup sliced fresh mushrooms
1 10.5-ounce package lite silken tofu
2 tablespoons prepared brown mustard
½ teaspoon nutritional yeast powder

½ teaspoon chili powder
¼ teaspoon dill weed
¼ teaspoon onion powder
¼ teaspoon garlic powder
¼ teaspoon turmeric
¼ teaspoon salt
several twists of freshly ground black pepper

Place the water in a medium nonstick frying pan. Add the onion, bell pepper, and mushrooms. Cook, stirring occasionally, for 5 minutes.

Meanwhile, place the tofu in a bowl and mash. Add the seasonings to the tofu and mix well. Add the tofu to the vegetables and cook for another 5 minutes, stirring frequently.

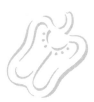

Recipe Hint: Serve with potatoes for a hearty breakfast. We also like this rolled up in a flour tortilla with salsa poured over the top. Refrigerate leftovers and use as a sandwich spread. We have prepared this for business breakfast meetings and watched traditional bacon-and-egg lovers going back for seconds.

Breakfast Banana Split

Servings: 2
Preparation Time:
10 minutes

2 bananas, sliced in half lengthwise
1 cup puffed wheat cereal
1 cup puffed rice cereal

1 8-ounce container nondairy vanilla yogurt
½ cup fresh blueberries
½ cup sliced fresh strawberries

Place 2 banana halves in each cereal bowl. Layer half of the ingredients in the order listed into 1 of the cereal bowls and repeat in the other bowl with the remaining ingredients.

STARCHES MAKE THE MEAL

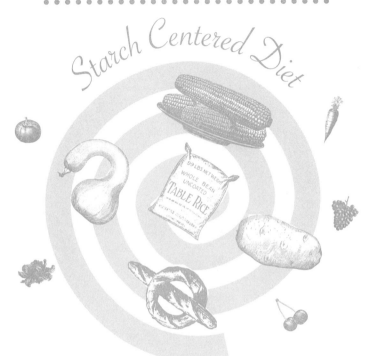

Starch Centered Diet

Many people are trying to eat healthier, but are failing. After bulking up on broccoli, cauliflower, and sprouts, they exclaim, "Nobody can eat this way." We agree: Nobody can eat a diet of green and yellow vegetables. They provide too few calories to be satisfying. The secret to a successful diet is to design it around delicious, satisfying starches. Everyone remembers these "comfort foods" that we loved growing up—potatoes, rice, pastas, corn, and beans: oatmeal, pancakes, and hash brown potatoes for breakfast; vegetable and bean soups for lunch; and spaghetti, bean burritos, and Spanish rice for dinner.

Starches are high in complex carbohydrates and dietary fiber, very low in fat, and contain no cholesterol. They are loaded with vitamins and minerals and always contain generous amounts of healthy vegetable protein that satisfies the nutritional needs of growing children and adults. Fruits and yellow and green vegetables are important additions to a starch-centered meal plan, providing a cornucopia of color, flavor, texture and aroma, as well as additional nutrients.

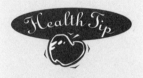

People look to supplements for better health, yet deficiency diseases like beriberi and scurvy are unknown in the United States. Our diseases are due to excesses—overindulgence in salt, sugar, protein, and cholesterol.

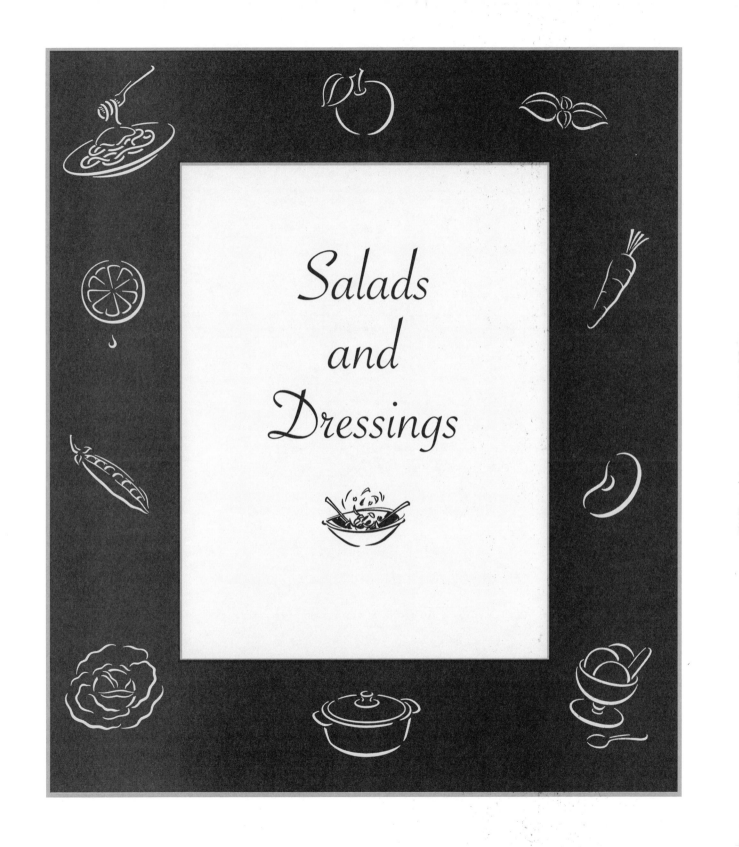

Salads
and
Dressings

Jicama Matchsticks

**1 medium jicama, peeled and
sliced into matchstick pieces**

⅛ cup lemon or lime juice
¼ teaspoon chili powder

Servings: 8
Preparation Time:
15 minutes

Place the jicama in a bowl with a lid. Add the juice and sprinkle the chili powder over the top. Cover and shake to distribute the seasonings. One of the women who works in our office very often carries this around with her in a small plastic container in case she gets hungry while she's away from home.

> **Recipe Hint:**   *To peel jicama, cut in half from top to bottom with a large knife. Place cut side down on a cutting board and cut off the brown skin in strips.*

Mexican Corn Salad

**4 cups frozen corn kernels,
thawed**
**1 15-ounce can black beans,
drained and rinsed**
½ cup chopped green onions

½ cup chopped red bell pepper
¼ cup chopped fresh cilantro
1 cup salsa
2 tablespoons balsamic vinegar

Servings: 6 to 8
Preparation Time:
15 minutes
Chilling Time:
2 hours

Combine the vegetables in a bowl. Place the salsa and vinegar in a blender jar and process until smooth. Pour over the vegetables and mix well. Refrigerate to blend the flavors.

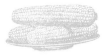

> **Recipe Hint:**   *To make this even spicier, add several dashes of Tabasco sauce when mixing the dressing into the vegetables.*

Servings: 5
Preparation Time:
15 minutes

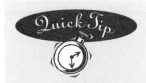

Triple-washed spinach is sold in bags in most supermarkets. It does not need to be washed again unless you wish to do so. Presliced mushrooms are also sold in packages.

Dijon Spinach Salad

1 10-ounce package triple-washed spinach
½ cup thinly sliced red onion, separated into rings

2 cups sliced fresh mushrooms
¾ cup Dijon-Oriental Dressing (page 48) *or* other oil-free salad dressing

Trim the spinach stems and tear into bite-size pieces. Add the onion and mushrooms and toss to mix. Pour the dressing over and toss again. Serve at once.

Simple Green Salad

Servings: 6
Preparation Time:
5 minutes

1 10-ounce package mixed washed greens
1 pint cherry tomatoes, halved

1 small burpless cucumber, cut in half lengthwise and thinly sliced

Combine all ingredients in a large bowl and toss to mix. Serve with your favorite oil-free salad dressing.

Washing all those spinach and salad leaves is a boring, time-consuming task. With packaged greens, you just cut them to desired size and use in salads, soups, and grain dishes.

Coleslaw

8 cups packaged coleslaw
  mix
1 carrot, shredded
½ cup chopped red onion

2 cups snow peas, cut in half
  crosswise (optional)
1 recipe Creamy Tofu Dressing
  (page 52)

*Servings: 6 to 8
Preparation Time:
5 minutes
(need prepared
Creamy Tofu Dressing)*

Combine all ingredients in a large bowl and toss well to mix. Serve at once or refrigerate until serving, up to 24 hours.

Thai Cabbage Salad

3½ tablespoons fresh lime juice
2 tablespoons soy sauce
½ to 1 teaspoon ground fresh
  chili paste

½ teaspoon minced fresh garlic
1 bag shredded cabbage
½ cup shredded carrot
green-leaf lettuce leaves

*Servings: 4
Preparation Time:
5 minutes*

Pour the lime juice and soy sauce in a small jar. Add the chili paste and garlic and shake well to mix. Set aside.

Place the shredded cabbage and carrot in a bowl. Mix well. Pour the dressing over the vegetables and toss to mix.

Serve on leaves of green-leaf lettuce.

Recipe Hint: *Ground fresh chili paste is also called Sambal Oelek. It can be found in most Asian markets. Shredded cabbage and shredded carrots are sold in bags in most supermarkets.*

CARBOHYDRATE SATISFIES

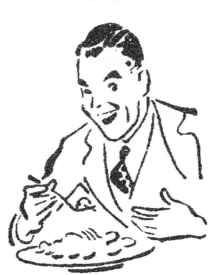

Carbohydrate =
Satisfaction

Fat =
NO Satisfaction

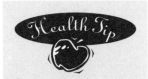

Starches, also called complex carbohydrates, are the most important foods for our bodies. They make us thin, not fat. Starches are familiar foods like beans, breads, corn, pastas, potatoes, and rice.

*E*ach of our drives to survive are satisfied by one specific thing. For example, the breathing drive is satisfied by oxygen. No other gas in the air will do. Thirst is satisfied only by water. And the hunger drive is satisfied by one component of our foods—carbohydrate. Fat does not satisfy our hunger.

The typical American meal consists of carbohydrate-deficient foods. All meats, including beef, pork, chicken, turkey, fish, and shellfish, contain no carbohydrate. Only 2 percent of the calories from cheese are carbohydrate. Lard, butter, olive oil, and corn oil contain no carbohydrate. John remembers eating these carbohydrate-deficient foods when he was growing up. After he finished his first plate, his body would say, "Johnny, that was interesting, but when are we going to eat?" After his second plate, his abdomen would distend slightly. Finally, after his third plate, the two signals came indicating he was done eating—he felt overstuffed and was in pain. He was still ravenously hungry, however, and if he could have found room for one more pork chop he would have stuffed it in.

Eating carbohydrate-rich starches, vegetables, and fruits will satisfy your hunger and free you from constant preoccupation with thoughts of food and the compulsive overeating that results. Now you can look great and never be hungry again!

Chinese Lettuce Salad

1 cup torn leaf lettuce
1 cup torn Chinese cabbage
1 cup fresh mung bean sprouts
½ cup sliced fresh mushrooms
½ cup snow peas

½ cup thinly sliced baby bok choy
½ cup chopped broccoli
⅔ cup Oriental Salad Dressing (page 48)

Combine the vegetables in a large bowl. Pour the dressing over and toss well to mix. Serve at once.

Servings: 4
Preparation Time: 15 minutes

Corn Salad

2 cups frozen corn kernels, thawed
1 red or green bell pepper, chopped
1 stalk celery, sliced

2 green onions, chopped
¼ cup sliced black olives
¼ cup sliced green olives
⅓ cup oil-free salad dressing

Combine all ingredients in a bowl and toss well to mix. Refrigerate for 1 hour to blend the flavors.

Recipe Hint: *To thaw corn quickly, place in a colander and hold under cold running water. Drain well before using.*

Servings: 4
Preparation Time: 10 minutes
Chilling Time: 1 hour

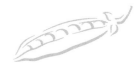

Potato Salad

Servings: 4
Preparation Time:
15 minutes
Cooking Time:
20 minutes

2 pounds small red potatoes, cut
   into chunks
½ cup finely chopped onion

½ cup finely chopped celery
½ cup chopped green onions

Dressing:

½ cup fat-free mayonnaise or
   Tofu Mayonnaise (page 255)
1 tablespoon prepared mustard
1 tablespoon soy or rice milk
1 tablespoon parsley flakes

½ teaspoon honey
¼ teaspoon dill weed
⅛ teaspoon salt
several twists of freshly ground
   black pepper

Place the potatoes in a pot with water to cover. Bring to a boil, cover, and cook over medium heat until just tender, about 20 minutes. (Don't let them get too soft.)

Meanwhile, combine all ingredients for the dressing in a bowl. Set aside.

When the potatoes are done, remove from heat and drain. Add the onion, celery, and green onions.

Pour the dressing over the vegetables and mix well. Serve warm or refrigerate up to 24 hours before serving.

Recipe Hint: Mary sometimes adds chopped cucumber, chopped radishes, and grated carrot to this salad. The dressing is our family's favorite for potato salad. If you have more than 6 cups of vegetable mixture, you may need to increase the dressing measurements accordingly; for example, for 1½ cups more vegetables, increase the dressing by one fourth, for 3 cups more vegetables, increase the dressing by one half, etc.

Garbanzo Zip Salad

1 15-ounce can garbanzo beans,
   drained and rinsed
1 tablespoon finely chopped
   onion

2 tablespoons finely chopped
   cilantro
¼ cup oil-free salad dressing

Servings: 1 to 2
Preparation Time:
5 minutes

Combine all ingredients in a bowl. Enjoy at room temperature or chill before serving, if desired.

Southwestern Bean Salad

1 15-ounce can black beans,
   drained and rinsed
1 15-ounce can corn, drained and
   rinsed
1 red bell pepper, chopped
1 bunch green onions, chopped

1 small bunch cilantro, chopped
½ cup balsamic vinegar
½ cup salsa
1 teaspoon minced fresh garlic
1 teaspoon ground cumin

Servings: 4
Preparation Time:
15 minutes
Chilling Time:
30 minutes

Combine the beans, corn, bell pepper, green onions, and cilantro in a bowl. Set aside. Combine the vinegar, salsa, garlic, and cumin and pour over the vegetables. Mix well. Chill for at least 30 minutes. Serve on a bed of finely shredded cabbage with baked tortilla chips.

Recipe Hint: *Chop the cilantro in a food processor to save time. Buy shredded cabbage in a bag. This salad tastes best when chilled overnight.*

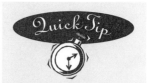

Keep a variety of oil-free salad dressings in your pantry. They can be used over packaged torn lettuce leaves for a quick green salad. They are also a delicious topping for baked potatoes, or use them to sauté vegetables.

Honey Bean Salad

Servings: 6 to 8
Preparation Time:
10 minutes
Chilling Time:
2 hours

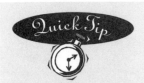

To thaw frozen vegetables quickly, place in a colander and hold under cold running water. Shake off excess water before using.

1 15-ounce can cut green beans, drained and rinsed
1 15-ounce can black beans, drained and rinsed
1 15-ounce can kidney beans, drained and rinsed
1 15-ounce can white beans, drained and rinsed

1½ cups frozen corn kernels, thawed
1 small red onion, thinly sliced and separated into rings
¼ cup oil-free honey mustard dressing
1 teaspoon chili powder

Combine all the vegetables in a large bowl. Pour the dressing over and sprinkle on the chili powder. Toss to mix. Refrigerate at least 2 hours for the flavors to blend.

Greek Salad

Servings: 6 to 8
Preparation Time:
15 minutes

4 to 5 large vine-ripened tomatoes, cut into small wedges
1 medium green bell pepper, coarsely chopped
1 small onion, sliced and separated into rings

1 cucumber, thinly sliced
¼ cup whole ripe olives (optional)
1 to 2 teaspoons finely chopped fresh oregano
½ cup oil-free Italian dressing

Combine all ingredients in a bowl. Toss to mix well. Serve at once or cover and chill until serving time.

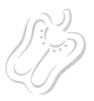

Recipe Hint: *In the summer of 1995 this salad was often the only vegetarian food we could find while traveling through Greece. "What kind of a salad will we get today?" became the family joke. We find this a very refreshing salad in the middle of the summer, with fresh, vine-ripened tomatoes. Make your Greek salad with your favorite cold sliced vegetables and oil-free salad dressing.*

THE FAT YOU EAT . . .
IS THE FAT YOU WEAR

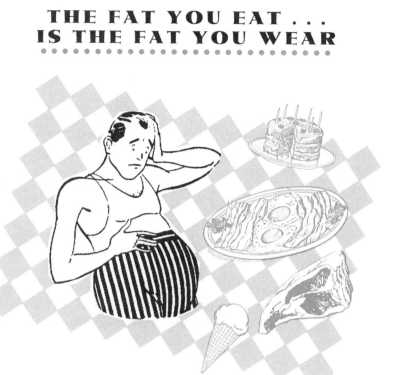

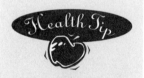

The body is efficient. Wasteful pathways for utilizing and disposing of excess nutrients are avoided. The proteins in our foods are used to repair cells and synthesize enzymes. Protein taken in excess is eliminated from the body through the kidneys. Excess protein is not stored or routinely converted into carbohydrate or fat. Carbohydrate is the body's main fuel. When more is consumed than is needed for daily activities, two pounds of the excess is stored invisibly in the liver and muscles as glycogen. The rest is dissipated as heat. The body does not turn extra carbohydrate into fat because the process is too wasteful.

Fats taken in excess of daily needs are also handled adeptly. Since they are already in the chemical form for storage, they are simply moved from the fork and spoon to the fat cells. The process is so efficient that the fats retain their original chemical structure. A needle biopsy of your fatty tissue would reveal the kinds of foods you like. If you eat lots of cold-water marine fish, then your fatty tissues will be full of omega-3 fats. If you like margarine, you will be full of "trans" fats. The fat you eat is the fat you wear. Effortlessly!

Health Tip

Fat is a general term for lipids that are solid at room temperature. They are usually from animal sources. Oils are liquid at room temperature and usually from plants or fish. In amounts commonly consumed, both fats and oils make people fat and sick.

Chili Bean Salad

Servings: 8
Preparation Time:
15 minutes
Chilling Time:
1 hour

1 15-ounce can garbanzo beans, drained and rinsed
1 15-ounce can kidney beans, drained and rinsed
1 15-ounce can white beans, drained and rinsed

1½ cup frozen corn kernels, thawed
1 red bell pepper, chopped
½ cup chopped green onions
1 4-ounce can chopped green chilies
⅓ cup chopped fresh cilantro

Dressing:

½ cup salsa
½ teaspoon chili powder

¼ teaspoon ground cumin

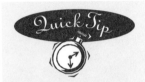

Have your refrigerator and pantry well stocked with salad dressings, barbecue sauces, steak sauces, salsas, and dried spices to add pizzazz to simple dishes in a hurry.

Combine all the vegetables in a large bowl. Mix the dressing ingredients together using a whisk. Pour the dressing over the vegetables and mix well. Refrigerate to blend the flavors.

Italian Bread Salad

Servings: 4
Preparation Time:
15 minutes

1 15-ounce can kidney beans, drained and rinsed
1 15-ounce can garbanzo beans, drained and rinsed
1 15-ounce can green beans, drained and rinsed

4 cups chopped tomatoes
4 cups cubed dense Italian-style oil-free bread
1 red onion, chopped
¾ cup oil-free Italian dressing
1 teaspoon dried basil

Combine all ingredients in a large bowl and toss well to mix.

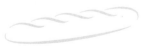

Barbecue Bean Salad

2 15-ounce cans small red beans,
    drained and rinsed
2 cups frozen corn kernels,
    thawed
1 green bell pepper, chopped

1 onion, chopped
⅓ cup oil-free honey Dijon-style
    salad dressing
¼ cup barbecue sauce

Servings: 4
Preparation Time:
10 minutes

Combine all ingredients in a bowl and toss well to mix. Serve at once or refrigerate until serving time.

Garden Bean Salad

2 15-ounce cans white beans,
    drained and rinsed
1 15-ounce can kidney beans,
    drained and rinsed
1 15-ounce can cut green beans,
    drained and rinsed

1 cup frozen corn kernels,
    thawed
1 green bell pepper, cut into
    strips
6 green onions, chopped
½ cup oil-free dill-cilantro salad
    dressing

Servings: 4
Preparation Time:
10 minutes

Combine all ingredients in a bowl and mix well. Serve at once or refrigerate for later use.

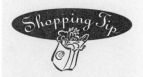

Shopping Tip

Make a list of all the items you buy regularly, leaving space to add extra items. Have it copied to serve as a starting list each week. Keep the list handy so you can add extra items for your next shopping trip.

Marinated Bean Salad

Servings: 4
Preparation Time:
15 minutes
Marinating Time:
1 hour

1 15-ounce can cooked white
   beans, drained and rinsed
1 cucumber, thinly sliced
¾ cup oil-free salad dressing
1 tomato, chopped

½ cup chopped green bell pepper
½ cup frozen corn kernels,
   thawed
2 teaspoons capers
4 large butter lettuce leaves

Combine the beans and cucumber in a bowl. Pour the dressing over and toss well to mix. Cover, place in the refrigerator, and let marinate for 1 hour.

After marinating, add the tomato, bell pepper, corn, and capers. Toss well to coat. Place 1 lettuce leaf on each of 4 plates and mound the vegetable mixture on the leaves. Serve at once.

Italian Potato and Bean Salad

Servings: 4
Preparation Time:
10 minutes
Chilling Time:
2 hours

1 16-ounce can sliced potatoes,
   drained and rinsed
1 15-ounce can garbanzo beans,
   drained and rinsed
1 stalk celery, sliced

4 green onions, chopped
¼ cup sliced black olives
⅓ cup oil-free Italian dressing
½ cup chopped tomatoes

Combine the potatoes, beans, celery, green onions, and olives in a bowl. Pour the dressing over and mix gently to coat. Cover and chill for 2 hours. Stir in the tomatoes just before serving.

CALORIE CONCENTRATION

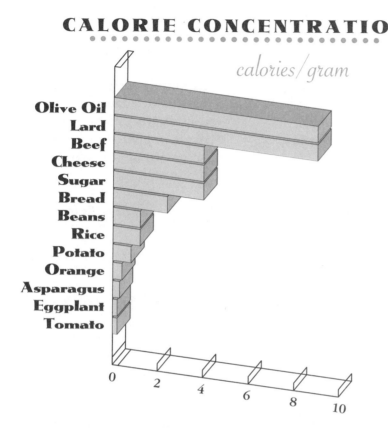

calories/gram

Olive Oil
Lard
Beef
Cheese
Sugar
Bread
Beans
Rice
Potato
Orange
Asparagus
Eggplant
Tomato

0   2   4   6   8   10

octors, dietitians, and scientists think of food in terms of calories per gram (cal/g). Olive oil is 9 cal/g, just like lard. Beef, cheese, and white sugar are 4 cal/g. Bread is 2.4 cal/g. Common whole starches like beans, rice, and potatoes are about 1 cal/g. Fruits and green and yellow vegetables are just a few tenths of a calorie per gram. When you change from the rich American diet to a starch-based diet you change the concentration of calories fourfold. In other words, for the same volume of food, the McDougall diet has one-quarter as many calories.

The "health food" olive oil is actually two and a half times more concentrated than "killer" white sugar. Olive oil is 100 percent fat; there is no carbohydrate in olive oil to satisfy hunger. White sugar contains no fat, so its extra calories will not be stored easily, and it is 100 percent carbohydrate, thereby providing great hunger satisfaction. So which is worse? Sprinkling a teaspoon of sugar on your cornflakes or dipping your bread in olive oil at the dinner table? There's a lot of truth to the saying "From my lips to my hips."

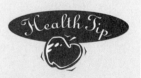

Fiber consists of microscopic chains of undigestible carbohydrate; it is not rough like the bristles of a broom. Fiber helps satisfy your appetite, encouraging weight loss by providing bulk with no calories.

White Bean Salad

Servings: 4 to 6
Preparation Time:
10 minutes
Chilling Time:
2 hours

2 15-ounce cans white beans, drained and rinsed
⅓ cup fresh lemon juice
½ teaspoon ground cumin
2 tomatoes, chopped
6 green onions, chopped
¼ cup finely chopped fresh parsley or cilantro
several twists of freshly ground black pepper
dash or two of Tabasco sauce

Combine all ingredients in a bowl and toss to mix. Refrigerate for 2 hours to blend flavors.

Asian Rice Salad

Servings: 4
Preparation Time:
15 minutes
(need cooked rice)
Chilling Time:
1 hour

2 cups cooked brown rice
4 green onions, chopped
5 cups loosely packed chopped spinach
1 11-ounce can mandarin orange segments, drained
1 8-ounce can sliced water chestnuts, drained
½ cup oil-free Dijon-style salad dressing
2 tablespoons soy sauce
½ cup avocado chunks (optional)

Place the rice in a large bowl. Add the green onions and spinach. Mix well. Add the orange segments and water chestnuts. Toss gently to mix.

Mix the dressing and soy sauce. Pour over the salad. Stir in the avocado, if desired. Cover and chill for 1 hour before serving.

Recipe Hint: *This salad should be served about 1 hour after preparing it. It becomes soggy after sitting for too long, although we have eaten some leftovers the next day and the flavor was still delicious.*

Southwestern Couscous Salad

Servings: 6
Preparation Time:
15 minutes

2 cups water
1¾ cups couscous
2 15-ounce cans black beans,
   drained and rinsed
2 cups frozen corn kernels,
   thawed

2 red bell peppers, chopped
1 tomato, chopped
½ cup chopped green onions
½ cup chopped cilantro
¾ cup Kozlowski Farms South of
   the Border Dressing

Bring the water to a boil. Add the couscous, stir, cover, remove from heat, and let rest for 10 minutes. Combine the couscous and vegetables. Pour the dressing over and toss to mix. Serve warm or cold.

Couscous (pasta) and bulgur (cracked grain) are quick to fix. Just soak them in boiling water for 10 minutes and they're ready to use to make tabouli, salads, and vegetable mixtures. Use them just as you would rice.

San Antonio Quinoa

Servings: 4
Preparation Time:
10 minutes
Cooking Time:
10 minutes
Chilling Time:
1 hour

1 cup vegetable broth
½ cup quinoa, rinsed
½ teaspoon cumin seed
1 15-ounce can black beans,
   drained and rinsed

1 cup frozen corn kernels, thawed
1 tomato, chopped
3 green onions, chopped
3 tablespoons chopped cilantro
½ cup oil-free dressing

Place the vegetable broth in a saucepan and bring to a boil. Add the quinoa and cumin. Cover, reduce heat, and simmer for 10 minutes. Remove from heat and set aside.

Combine the beans, corn, tomato, green onions, and cilantro in a bowl. Add the quinoa and dressing and toss well to mix. Refrigerate at least 1 hour before serving.

Recipe Hint: Vary the dressing to suit your taste. We have even used salsa on several occasions with good results. Quinoa (pronounced keen-wa) is a high-protein grain. Uncooked, it looks somewhat like toasted sesame seeds. It becomes translucent when cooked. It is available in natural food stores.

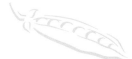

Bulgur and Corn Salad

Servings: 4
Preparation Time:
10 minutes
Soaking Time:
15 minutes
Chilling Time:
1 hour (optional)

2 cups boiling water
1 cup uncooked bulgur
1 cup frozen corn kernels,
    thawed
¼ cup finely chopped red onion

⅛ cup chopped fresh cilantro
¼ cup Oriental Salad Dressing
    (page 48) or other oil-free
    dressing

Pour the boiling water over the bulgur, cover, and let rest for 15 minutes.

Meanwhile, combine the corn, onion, and cilantro in a separate bowl.

After 15 minutes, drain the bulgur and fluff with a fork. Add to the vegetables and mix well. Pour the dressing over and toss to coat. Refrigerate before serving, if desired.

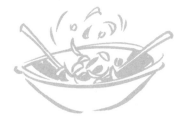

EAT AND LOSE WEIGHT

For Overweight People: 1,088 patients

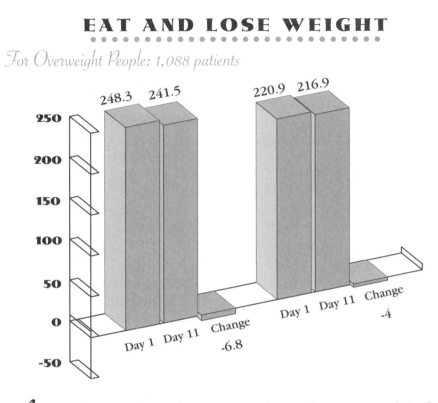

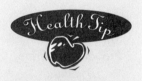

At our clinic at St. Helena Hospital people are served "cafeteria style" from a buffet table. They eat as much as they want, just as they do at home. Yet, the average weight loss for overweight men (starting over 200 pounds) is 6.8 pounds and overweight women (starting over 175 pounds) is 4 pounds in eleven days; while they stuff themselves with four-course, chef-prepared gourmet meals. Typical meals are oatmeal, home fried potatoes, pancakes, toast, and fruit for breakfast; spaghetti, grain and bean burgers, soups, and salads for lunch; and stuffed squash, lasagne, Chinese stir-fry, soups, and salads for dinner. The food is so well prepared that everyone loves it from the first day.

The hunger drive is unbeatably strong. That's why we encourage people to eat. "The more you eat the thinner and healthier you will become," we tell them. Of course, you must eat the right foods. The program also includes daily exercise, which burns calories, regulates the appetite, and builds calorie-burning muscle tissue. For faster and greater weight loss, exercise more; and modify the basic McDougall diet to eliminate flour products (breads, bagels, and pastas), and increase your intake of rice, corn, potatoes, and green and yellow vegetables.

Health Tip

Eating healthy is simply learning to like new foods. Finding time to exercise is simply a matter of just saying, "Yes, I will take the time to exercise today." Most importantly, find an exercise you like, so you'll stay with it.

Couscous Tabouli

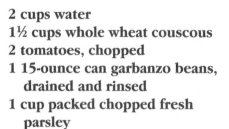

Servings: 8
Preparation Time:
15 minutes
Cooking Time:
5 minutes

2 cups water
1½ cups whole wheat couscous
2 tomatoes, chopped
1 15-ounce can garbanzo beans, drained and rinsed
1 cup packed chopped fresh parsley

½ cup packed chopped fresh mint
6 green onions, thinly sliced
½ cup fresh lemon juice
freshly ground black pepper to taste

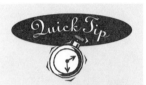

To chop parsley quickly, place sprigs in a large measuring cup and cut with kitchen shears.

Bring the water to a boil. Remove from heat and add the couscous. Stir, cover, and let rest for 5 minutes. Fluff with a fork. Cool slightly by placing in a colander.

Combine the remaining ingredients, except the pepper, in a separate bowl. Add the couscous and mix well. Season with the pepper.

Serve at room temperature, or chill before serving.

Basmati Rice Salad

Servings: 4
Preparation Time:
10 minutes
(need cooked rice)

2 cups cooked basmati rice
1 16-ounce can corn, drained and rinsed
1 15-ounce can black beans, drained and rinsed
2 green onions, chopped

4 radishes, thinly sliced
⅓ cup lime juice
1 teaspoon ground cumin
cayenne pepper to taste
1 to 2 tablespoons chopped cilantro

Mix all the ingredients, except the cilantro, in a bowl. Eat at room temperature or heat for 3 to 4 minutes in a microwave, stirring once halfway through the cooking time. Sprinkle the cilantro on top before eating.

Confetti Salad

2 cups cooked brown rice
2 cups frozen corn kernels, thawed
1 tomato, coarsely chopped
½ cup chopped green pepper
½ cup chopped green onions
1 2.25-ounce can sliced black
   olives, drained

¼ cup chopped fresh dill weed
½ teaspoon Dijon-style mustard
2 tablespoons water
2 tablespoons wine vinegar
2 tablespoons soy sauce
several dashes of Tabasco
   sauce

Servings: 6 to 8
Preparation Time:
15 minutes
(need cooked rice)
Chilling Time:
2 hours

Mix the brown rice, corn, tomato, green pepper, green onions, olives, and dill in a large bowl. Set aside.

Place the mustard in a small jar. Add 1 tablespoon water and mix until it is smooth. Add the remaining 1 tablespoon water, the vinegar, soy sauce, and Tabasco. Mix well. Pour over the salad. Toss well to mix. Cover and chill for at least 2 hours before serving for the best flavor.

Recipe Hint: *If you're in a rush, this salad may also be served soon after mixing. It is wonderful to take to a picnic or potluck because everyone loves it.*

Quinoa Salad

Servings: 8 to 10
Preparation Time:
15 minutes
Cooking Time:
15 minutes
Chilling Time:
2 hours

1½ cups quinoa
3 cups water
1 green bell pepper, chopped
1 red bell pepper, chopped
½ cup green onions, chopped
½ cup chopped cucumber
½ cup chopped celery

1 2-ounce jar chopped
   pimiento
¼ cup finely chopped fresh dill,
   cilantro, or parsley
½ cup oil-free salad dressing
freshly ground black pepper to
   taste

Rinse the quinoa well before cooking to remove the slightly bitter coating. Place the quinoa and water in a saucepan, bring to a boil, cover, reduce heat, and simmer over low heat for about 15 minutes, until the liquid is absorbed.

Combine the chopped vegetables in a bowl, including the fresh chopped herb of your choice. Mix well. Add the cooked quinoa. Toss gently and add the dressing. Toss again and add the pepper. Cover and chill for at least 2 hours.

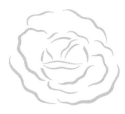

Rice and Lettuce Salad

Servings: 6
Preparation Time:
15 minutes
(need cooked rice)

4 cups cooked rice
6 cups packaged lettuce salad
1 15-ounce can kidney beans,
   drained and rinsed

1 15-ounce can black beans,
   drained and rinsed
1 cup oil-free salad dressing

To serve, place about ¾ cup of the rice on each of 6 plates. The rice may be either hot or cold. Spread 1 cup of the lettuce over the rice. Spoon some of each of the beans over the lettuce, then pour the dressing over the top.

Recipe Hint: *This is a fast, easy meal for those days when you are really rushed. It may sound strange to layer lettuce over hot rice, but it is delicious. Change the beans and dressing used to vary the salad.*

Hot Rice Salad

½ cup vegetable broth
2 bunches green onions, cut into
   1-inch pieces
1 stalk celery, sliced
1 red bell pepper, chopped
1 zucchini, chopped
1 cup broccoli florets
½ teaspoon minced garlic

1 tablespoon parsley flakes
½ teaspoon basil
½ teaspoon dill weed
½ teaspoon paprika
4 cups hot cooked brown rice
   (use instant brown rice or
   microwave-cooked rice)
1 tomato, chopped

Servings: 6
Preparation Time:
15 minutes
(need cooked rice)
Cooking Time:
10 minutes

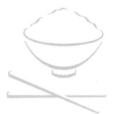

Place the broth in a large saucepan. Add the green onions, celery, bell pepper, zucchini, broccoli, and garlic. Cook, stirring occasionally, for 5 minutes. Add the seasonings. Cook for another 5 minutes. Remove from heat. Stir in the hot rice and tomato. Mix well and serve.

Recipe Hint: *Buy cleaned chopped broccoli in the supermarket to save time.*

CHANGE FOUNDATIONS

muscles   *starches*

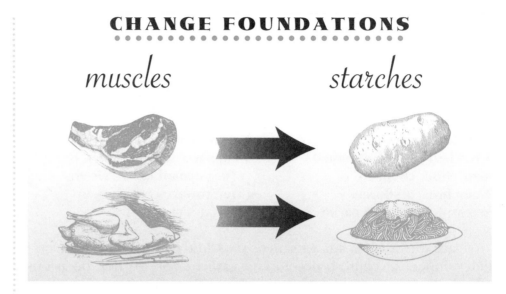

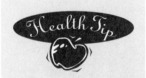

Only plant foods contain dietary fiber, and processing removes fiber. The American diet provides 10 grams of fiber a day. You're now eating 40 to 80 grams of fiber on the McDougall Program. The benefits will be seen first in your intestines.

When you were growing up, and someone asked "What's for dinner?" the usual response was "chicken," "steak," "pork chops," or "fish." The meat was the focus of the meal. Now when someone asks "What's for dinner?" your response will be "spaghetti," "bean burritos," "hash brown potatoes," or "spicy Spanish rice." Starch becomes the centerpiece of the meal.

A meat centerpiece for a meal is really rather tasteless—think about plain, unsalted, broiled or boiled chicken or beef. There is very little flavor. To make this bland meat interesting, you must cover it with a spicy tomato, sweet and sour, or barbecue sauce. As we all know, meats and dairy products are full of fat and cholesterol; they contain no dietary fiber or complex carbohydrate. They're unhealthy for us to eat.

You solve this dietary problem by substituting healthy (also rather tasteless) foods such as pasta, potatoes, and rice for the unhealthy, bland foods. Take your favorite sauces, make them healthy by removing any oil or animal products, and pour them over your newly chosen healthy centerpieces. This way all you give up is bad health—not a bit of good taste.

Lemon Couscous Salad

4 cups water
2 cups couscous
1 15-ounce can garbanzo beans, drained and rinsed
1 bunch green onions, chopped
1 cup finely chopped fresh spinach

1 2.25-ounce can sliced black olives, drained and rinsed
½ cup lemon juice
2 tablespoons fresh chopped parsley
¼ teaspoon garlic powder
¼ teaspoon dill weed

Servings: 8
Preparation Time: 15 minutes
Chilling Time: 1 to 2 hours

Place the water in a saucepan and bring to a boil. Add the couscous. Cook and stir for 1 minute. Turn off heat, cover, and let stand for 10 minutes. Combine the remaining ingredients in a bowl. Add the couscous and mix well. Chill for 1 to 2 hours before serving.

Recipe Hint: This salad may be eaten warm if you wish. We also like it without the spinach, so don't hesitate to make it if you don't have any spinach on hand. This salad tends to soak up the lemon juice. When there are leftovers, you may have to add a bit more lemon juice to moisten the salad the next day.

Aloha Rice Salad

Servings: 6
Preparation Time:
15 minutes
(need cooked rice)
Chilling Time:
2 hours

1 8-ounce can pineapple chunks
   in juice
3 cups cold cooked brown rice
1 red bell pepper, chopped

1 cup chopped cucumber
1 cup shredded carrots
½ cup chopped green onions

Dressing:

2 tablespoons lime juice
2 tablespoons sherry
2 tablespoons chopped fresh
   cilantro

1 tablespoon rice vinegar
1 teaspoon minced fresh
   gingerroot

Drain the pineapple, reserving 3 tablespoons of the juice in a separate bowl.

Mix the pineapple chunks, rice, and vegetables. Combine the dressing ingredients with the reserved pineapple juice. Pour the dressing over the salad and toss to mix. Refrigerate for at least 2 hours to blend the flavors.

Couscous Salad with Spicy Soy-Yogurt Dressing

1 onion, chopped
1 stalk celery, chopped

1 cup couscous
1¾ cups water

Servings: 4 to 6
Preparation Time:
15 minutes
Cooking Time:
5 minutes
Resting Time:
30 minutes

Dressing:

4 tablespoons plain nondairy
   yogurt
4 tablespoons lemon juice
2 teaspoons minced fresh
   gingerroot

1 teaspoon ground turmeric
½ teaspoon minced garlic
½ teaspoon ground cumin
½ teaspoon ground coriander

Optional toppings:

chopped green onions, chopped cilantro, garbanzo beans, chopped
   red bell pepper, currants

Place the onion and celery in a medium saucepan with ¼ cup of the water. Cook, stirring occasionally, until softened, about 3 minutes. Add the couscous and mix well. Stir in the remaining 1½ cups water. Bring to a boil, cover, and remove from heat. Let rest for 30 minutes.

Combine the dressing ingredients in a separate bowl. Chill while the couscous is resting.

To serve, fluff the couscous mixture with a fork. Add the desired toppings to the couscous and then spoon the dressing over the top.

Recipe Hint: *The dressing is also delicious on other salads or baked potatoes.*

Pastina

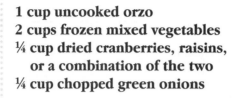

*Servings: 4 to 6
Preparation Time:
5 minutes
Cooking Time:
10 minutes
Chilling Time:
2 hours*

1 cup uncooked orzo
2 cups frozen mixed vegetables
¼ cup dried cranberries, raisins,
   or a combination of the two
¼ cup chopped green onions

½ cup oil-free honey Dijon
   dressing
1 tablespoon soy sauce
freshly ground black pepper to
   taste

Bring 4 cups of water to a boil. Add the orzo. Cook for 4 minutes, until the orzo is tender. Meanwhile, place the frozen vegetables in a glass bowl. Add ¼ cup water, cover, and microwave on high for 6 minutes.

Drain the orzo and vegetables. Combine the orzo, vegetables, dried fruit, and green onions. Mix the dressing and soy sauce. Pour over the orzo mixture and toss to mix. Season with the pepper. Refrigerate at least 2 hours to blend the flavors.

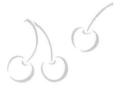

Recipe Hint: *This makes a wonderful side-dish salad with a soup meal. It is also ideal to take to work for an easy and delicious lunch. After chilling, we sometimes have to add a little more dressing to moisten this salad. The orzo just seems to soak up the dressing. This is also good with an oil-free Italian-style dressing.*

THE McDOUGALL "OIL EMBARGO"

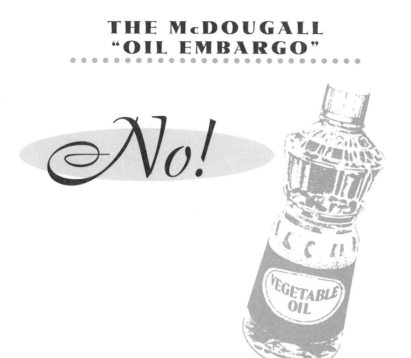

No!

The most unpalatable and unhealthy component of the American diet is grease—in other words, fats and oils. We wash our hands and face immediately when we get fats and oils on them. Strong detergents are used to remove repulsive grease from our countertops and walls. What do people call a restaurant with a bad reputation? A greasy spoon! The revulsion we feel toward grease is a way of protecting our health. The only way to make greasy foods palatable is to add salt, sugar, and spice to them—the more the better. One reason manufacturers use fats and oils is to get the ingredients we do like to stick to our foods. Oils stick the salt to the potato chips and French fries, the sugar to the donuts, and the spices to the salad leaves. Fortunately, there are healthy ways for salt, sugar, and spice to stick to foods without using disgusting, damaging fats and oils. We can easily remove grease from our diet by using nonstick cookware and healthy cooking and baking techniques. It's easy! And the food is even more delicious. The only thing you give up when you eliminate fats and oils is bad health.

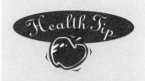

Health Tip

Plant foods naturally contain small amounts of fat. A nutritional label that lists 2 grams of fat, with no added oils listed in the ingredients, is referring to this natural, healthy fat.

Hot Pasta and Bean Salad

Servings: 8
Preparation Time:
5 minutes
Cooking Time:
15 minutes

1 pound rotini pasta
2 cups broccoli florets
1 pint cherry tomatoes, halved
1 15-ounce can garbanzo beans, drained and rinsed

1 15-ounce can black beans, drained and rinsed
1 15-ounce can kidney beans, drained and rinsed
¼ cup sliced black olives
½ cup oil-free Italian dressing

Cook the pasta according to package directions. Drain and set aside. While the pasta is cooking, place the broccoli in a glass bowl with ½ cup water. Cover and place in the microwave. Cook on high for about 4 minutes, until crisp-tender. Drain. Combine the broccoli, tomatoes, beans, and olives. Add the pasta and toss to mix. Add the dressing and mix again. Serve hot.

Recipe Hint: *Buy cut broccoli florets in bags in the supermarket to save time.*

Olé Pasta Salad

Servings: 8
Preparation Time:
15 minutes
Cooking Time:
10 minutes
Chilling Time:
2 hours

2 cups small uncooked pasta
1 15-ounce can kidney beans, drained and rinsed
1 red or green bell pepper, chopped
3 plum tomatoes, chopped

1 4-ounce can chopped green chilies
1 2.25-ounce can sliced black olives, drained and rinsed
⅓ cup oil-free Italian dressing
⅓ cup salsa

Place a large pot of water on to boil. Drop the pasta in the boiling water and cook, uncovered, until al dente, tender but still firm. Drain and rinse under cold water.

Combine the remaining ingredients in a large bowl. Add the cooked pasta and toss well to mix. Refrigerate for 2 hours to blend the flavors.

California Pasta Salad

1 12-ounce bag medium-size
  pasta
1 16-ounce bag frozen California
  blend vegetables (broccoli,
  cauliflower, carrots)

1 cup oil-free Italian
  dressing

Servings: 6 to 8
Preparation Time:
5 minutes
Cooking Time:
10 minutes

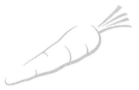

    Bring water to a boil, drop in the pasta, and cook according to package directions. Pour the frozen vegetables in a colander to thaw while the pasta is cooking. When the pasta has finished cooking, pour it and the cooking water over the vegetables in the colander. Let rest for a few minutes. Pour into a bowl, add the dressing, and toss well to mix. Serve warm or cold.

> **Recipe Hint:** *This is a very easy, fast pasta salad that can be varied. Change the shape of the pasta, use different combinations of frozen vegetables (many choices are available in 16-ounce bags in every supermarket), and use different oil-free salad dressings.*

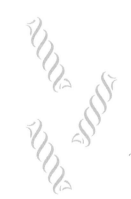

Garden Pasta Salad

Servings: 6 to 8
Preparation Time:
15 minutes
Cooking Time:
10 minutes
Chilling Time:
2 hours

1 12-ounce package rainbow pasta
1 16-ounce package frozen chopped mixed vegetables, thawed
1 cup sliced fresh mushrooms

3 green onions, thinly sliced
1 2-ounce jar chopped pimientos
½ cup cherry tomatoes, halved
1 cup oil-free Italian dressing freshly ground black pepper to taste

Bring 4 quarts of water to a boil, add the pasta, and cook according to package directions. Drain. Rinse under cool water and set aside.

Combine the pasta and the remaining ingredients in a large bowl. Toss to mix well. Refrigerate at least 2 hours before serving.

Recipe Hint: Use interesting vegetable combinations, such as broccoli and cauliflower; broccoli, corn, and red pepper; or broccoli, red pepper, snap peas, and water chestnuts.

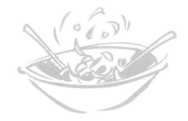

Thai Noodle Salad

1 10-ounce package Chinese
  noodles
⅓ cup rice vinegar
3 tablespoons soy sauce
3 tablespoons lime juice
3 tablespoons sugar

1 teaspoon minced fresh garlic
1 teaspoon ground fresh chili
  paste
dash of sesame oil (optional)
¾ cup shredded carrot
¾ cup chopped cilantro

Servings: 8 to 10
Preparation Time:
10 minutes
Cooking Time:
3 minutes

Bring 6 quarts of water to a boil. Drop in the noodles. Cook until tender, about 3 minutes, stirring constantly to separate the noodles. Pour into a colander and rinse with cold water.

Combine the remaining ingredients, except the carrot and cilantro, in a large bowl. Stir to mix and dissolve the sugar. Add the noodles, carrot, and cilantro. Toss to mix. Serve immediately or chill up to 4 hours.

Recipe Hint: *The brand of Chinese noodles that we use is called China Bowl Select. They are made from wheat flour, pea flour, and salt. Other brands may be substituted, but make sure they do not contain eggs or oil. Ground fresh chili paste is also called Sambal Oelek. It can be found in most Asian markets. Shredded carrots can be purchased in bags in some supermarkets.*

PROTEIN IS PLENTIFUL

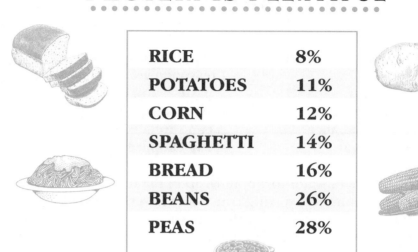

RICE	8%
POTATOES	11%
CORN	12%
SPAGHETTI	14%
BREAD	16%
BEANS	26%
PEAS	28%

A protein deficient diet is impossible!

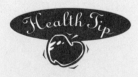

Protein is so abundant in plant foods that it is impossible to design a diet based on starches and vegetables that fails to provide for the needs of children and adults. Problems with protein are too much, not too little.

Experimental studies carried out in the 1940s and 1950s showed that people require about 2.5 percent of their calories as protein. In order to provide a definitely safe level—to cover situations such as chronic infection and injuries—the World Health Organization (WHO) doubled these figures. Since 1974, WHO has recommended that men, women, and children consume about 5 percent of their calories as protein. Pregnant women should consume about 6.5 percent of their calories as protein, and lactating women 7 percent.

Nature designed her foods to be complete long before they arrived on the dinner table. Think about it. There is sufficient protein in plants to grow elephants, horses, and hippos, so there ought to be enough to grow human beings. The most rapid time of growth in a person's life is during infancy. We double in size in the first two years of life. No one would contest that the ideal food for a baby is human breast milk, which is only 5 percent protein. Commonly consumed starches and vegetables contain from 6 to 45 percent of their calories as protein, and therefore are more than sufficient to supply the protein needs of children and adults, who grow at a much slower rate than babies.

Island Salad

4 cups torn lettuce leaves
1 avocado, peeled and
    diced
1 mango, peeled and diced

½ small red onion, thinly sliced
    and separated into rings
½ cup oil-free cilantro-dill
    dressing

Servings: 2
Preparation Time:
10 minutes

Combine the vegetables and fruit in a bowl. Pour the dressing over and toss to mix.

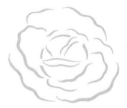

Recipe Hint: *You can change the flavor of the salad by changing the kind of dressing used. Many oil-free, dairy-free dressings are sold in supermarkets. Try some of the oil-free dressings in this book (pages 48–52). Substitute papaya for the mango.*

Tropical Fruit Salad

½ honeydew melon, peeled,
    seeded, and cubed
1 papaya, peeled, seeded, and
    cubed
1 mango, peeled, cut away from
    the pit, and chopped

1 pint strawberries, stemmed and
    halved
1 8-ounce can pineapple chunks,
    drained

Servings: 6
Preparation Time:
15 minutes

Combine all ingredients in a bowl and toss well to mix. Serve drizzled with lime juice or with Chili Citrus Dressing (page 51).

Recipe Hint: *Vary this salad by changing the fruit to whatever is available in your area. Try it with cantaloupe, watermelon, peaches, and halved grapes. Blueberries and raspberries also make nice additions.*

Spicy Salad Dressing

*Servings: makes
1½ cups
Preparation Time:
5 minutes*

¾ cup rice or wine vinegar
½ cup soy sauce
3 tablespoons sugar
2 tablespoons minced fresh
   gingerroot

1½ teaspoons minced fresh
   garlic
1 to 2 teaspoons crushed red
   pepper

Combine all ingredients in a jar and shake to mix.

Recipe Hint: To thicken this dressing, add ¼ teaspoon of guar gum to the mixture before shaking. Guar gum is a thickening agent that does not require cooking. Shake well and refrigerate for 1 hour. This is excellent on grain, bean, or vegetable salads.

Oriental Salad Dressing

*Servings: makes
¾ cup
Preparation Time:
5 minutes*

¼ cup soy sauce
¼ cup rice vinegar
¼ cup water

¼ teaspoon minced fresh garlic
¼ teaspoon minced fresh
   gingerroot

Combine all ingredients in a blender jar and process until smooth. Store in a covered jar in the refrigerator.

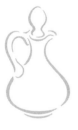

Recipe Hint: To make this into a Dijon-Oriental dressing, add 2 teaspoons Dijon-style mustard to the ingredients before processing.

Vinaigrette Dressing

3 tablespoons plain nondairy
   yogurt
3 tablespoons orange juice
3 tablespoons chopped fresh
   cilantro or parsley
2 tablespoons water

2 tablespoons white wine vinegar
2 tablespoons lime juice
1 tablespoon sugar
1 teaspoon chili powder
½ teaspoon onion powder
½ teaspoon ground cumin

*Servings: makes
¾ cup
Preparation Time:
5 minutes*

Combine all ingredients in a covered jar. Shake to mix. Use at once or refrigerate for later use.

Recipe Hint: *Nondairy yogurt is made from soy milk and is available in plain and fruit-flavored varieties. It is sold in natural food stores.*

Creamy Cilantro-Garlic Dressing

2 cups cilantro leaves
1 teaspoon minced fresh
   garlic
⅛ cup water

1 10.5-ounce package lite silken
   tofu
1 tablespoon lemon juice
1 tablespoon soy sauce

*Servings: makes
1½ cups
Preparation Time:
10 minutes
Chilling Time:
2 hours*

Place the cilantro, garlic, and water in a food processor. Process until blended. Add the remaining ingredients and process until smooth. Chill for at least 2 hours before using.

Recipe Hint: *Serve as a dip for vegetables as well as a dressing for salads. To vary, use 1 cup parsley and 1 cup cilantro. Try balsamic vinegar instead of lemon juice. You can also use fresh basil leaves. Omit the lemon juice when using basil.*

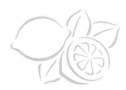

COMPLETE PROTEIN

Grams/Day	Min.	Recom.	Corn	Rice	Wheat	Potato
Tryptophan	.25	.50	.66	.71	1.4	.8
Phenylalanine	.28	.56	6.13	3.1	5.9	3.6
Leucine	1.10	2.20	12.0	5.5	8.0	4.1
Isoleucine	.7	1.4	4.1	3.0	5.2	3.6
Lysine	.8	1.6	4.1	2.5	3.2	4.4
Valine	.8	1.6	6.8	4.5	5.5	4.4
Methionine	.11	.22	2.1	1.1	1.8	1.0
Threonine	.5	1.0	4.5	2.5	3.5	3.4
Total Protein	20.0	37.0	109.0	64.0	120.0	82.0

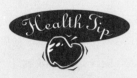

Health Tip

Hunger is satisfied by single foods, such as rice or potatoes. We have no drive to cause us to mix foods to make "complete proteins." Now there is strong evidence combining foods for better nutrition is completely unnecessary.

The building blocks of protein are twenty amino acids. The proteins of whales, elm trees, viruses, and other living things are all made of the same twenty amino acids arranged in different sequences—just as all the words in a dictionary are made of the same twenty-six letters of the alphabet. Humans can make twelve of these amino acids; therefore, these are called the *unessential* amino acids, because they don't have to be in our foods. The eight amino acids that we cannot synthesize are *essential* amino acids we must get from our foods.

Scientific studies determined both the minimum amino acid requirement and a value twice as great, referred to as the "recommended" or "definitely safe" level. Comparing the amounts of essential amino acids supplied by single foods demonstrates how every starch and vegetable supplies each of the essential amino acids in excess of the recommended, "definitely safe" level. It is impossible to design a diet based on unprocessed starches and vegetables that fails to provide for the essential amino acid requirements of children or adults.

Tofu Island Dressing

1 10.5-ounce package lite silken tofu
1 tablespoon lemon juice
3 tablespoons ketchup
2 tablespoons sweet pickle relish

1 tablespoon minced parsley
1 tablespoon minced red onion
1 teaspoon soy sauce
several twists of freshly ground black pepper

Servings: 1½ cups
Preparation Time:
5 minutes
Chilling Time:
2 hours

Place the tofu and lemon juice in a blender or food processor and process until smooth. Place in a bowl and stir in the remaining ingredients. Chill for at least 2 hours before using.

Recipe Hint: *This thick salad dressing is similar to Thousand Island dressing.*

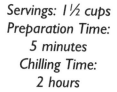

Chili Citrus Dressing

⅓ cup orange juice
3 tablespoons lime juice
3 tablespoons fresh cilantro, parsley, or basil

2 tablespoons chopped canned green chilies
1 tablespoon honey

Servings: makes
¾ cup
Preparation Time:
5 minutes

Combine all ingredients in a blender and process until well blended. Serve over fruit salads.

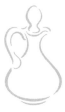

Creamy Tofu Dressing

Servings: 1½ cups
Preparation Time:
5 minutes
Chilling Time:
2 hours

1 10.5-ounce package lite silken
  tofu
2 tablespoons balsamic vinegar
1 tablespoon honey
1 teaspoon prepared horseradish

¼ teaspoon garlic powder
¼ teaspoon salt
⅛ teaspoon dry mustard
several twists of freshly ground
  black pepper

Combine all ingredients in a blender or food processor and process until smooth. Adjust the thickness of the dressing to your liking by adding small amounts of water and processing until it is the desired consistency. Chill for at least 2 hours before using.

Recipe Hint: Use this as a replacement for mayonnaise. It is good on sandwiches or as a dressing for coleslaw. To use as a salad dressing, thin as directed above with a small amount of water. Any dressing or spread made with tofu is best prepared about a day ahead of time so that the flavors can blend to give you the best results. Most dressings made with tofu keep in the refrigerator for about 1 week.

Soups
and
Stews

Quick Vegetable Broth

8 cups water
1 onion, chopped
3 cups coarsely chopped assorted
  vegetables

¼ cup fresh parsley leaves
1 bay leaf
several twists of freshly ground
  black pepper

Combine all ingredients in a large pot. Bring to a boil over high heat. Skim off any foam, reduce heat, and simmer for 30 minutes. Strain into another pot. Push on the vegetables with a large spoon to extract as much juice as possible. Discard the vegetables. Store in the refrigerator for 3 days or freeze for up to 3 months.

Recipe Hint: We usually make this in our pasta pot, which has a liner with holes in it like a colander. We cut the vegetables in large pieces so that they will not fit through the holes. After cooking, we just have to lift the basket out of the pot and push on the vegetables with a spoon to extract the liquids. Use whatever vegetables you have in your refrigerator: carrots, celery, mushroom stems, broccoli stalks, pea pods, cauliflower stalks, zucchini ends, spinach stems, parsley stems, etc.

*Servings: makes
4 cups
Preparation Time:
15 minutes
Cooking Time:
30 minutes*

The vegetable section of your supermarket has carrots, celery, broccoli, and cauliflower precut for your convenience. Use them raw to make salads or cook for side dishes. Add during cooking to make quick and easy soups and stews. Frozen vegetables are usually partially cooked.

Broccoli Pasta Soup

8 cups vegetable broth
4 cups broccoli florets
½ pound uncooked pasta
  (shells, rotini, broken
  linguine)

1 tablespoon soy sauce
dash of Tabasco sauce
  (optional)

*Servings: 8
Preparation Time:
5 minutes
Cooking Time:
30 minutes*

Place the broth in a large soup pot and bring to a boil. Add the pasta and cook for about 5 to 6 minutes, until it is almost done. Add the remaining ingredients, mix well, and turn off heat. Cover and let rest for 20 minutes. Serve with some fresh bread to dunk in the broth.

Cream of Celery Soup

Servings: 4
Preparation Time:
   15 minutes
Cooking Time:
   15 minutes

1 onion, chopped
5 ribs celery, chopped
⅔ cup water
3 tablespoons unbleached white
   flour

1¾ cups vegetable broth
1½ cups rice milk
1 tablespoon soy sauce
several twists of freshly ground
   black pepper

Place the onion and celery in a pot with the water. Cook until soft, about 10 minutes. Stir in the flour and mix well. Add the remaining ingredients. Bring to a boil, reduce heat, and cook gently for 5 minutes. Remove 2 cups of the soup from the pot and place in a blender. Puree, return to the pot, and mix well. Serve at once.

Recipe Hint: Chop the onion and celery in a food processor to save time. This soup is almost always a favorite with children.

Taco Soup

Servings: 4
Preparation Time:
   10 minutes
Cooking Time:
   10 minutes

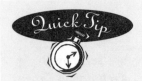

To prepare the avocado, cut it lengthwise and twist the halves in opposite directions to separate. Hit the seed with a sharp knife hard enough so that the knife sticks into it. Twist the knife and remove the seed.

3½ cups vegetable broth
1 15-ounce can black beans,
   drained and rinsed
1¼ cups chunky mild or medium-
   hot salsa

1¼ cups frozen corn
   kernels
1 cup avocado chunks
1 cup fat-free tortilla chips

Place the broth, beans, salsa, and corn in a medium saucepan. Cook over low heat for 10 minutes to blend the flavors.

Meanwhile, chop the avocado and break up the chips into bite-size pieces. To serve, place one quarter of the avocado and chips in the bottom of 4 serving bowls. Ladle the soup over the avocado and chips and serve at once.

LOWER YOUR BLOOD PRESSURE

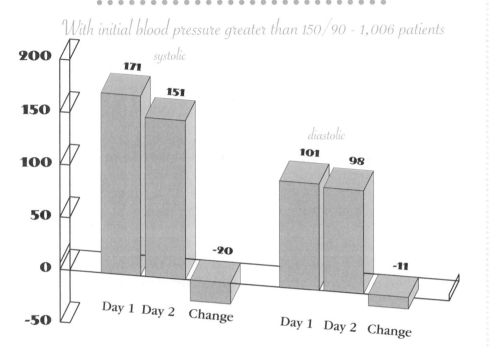

With initial blood pressure greater than 150/90 - 1,006 patients

systolic

171 151 -20

diastolic

101 98 -11

200 150 100 50 0 -50

Day 1 Day 2 Change   Day 1 Day 2 Change

*A*t least one in three adults in the United States has elevated blood pressure. A normal blood pressure is 110/70 or less for a person who does not take blood pressure-lowering medications. This value is associated with the lowest risk of health problems. As your blood pressure rises, your likelihood of suffering a heart attack or stroke increases.

Blood pressures of our patients fall quickly for several reasons: They're relaxed at St. Helena Hospital in the Napa Valley, California. They're off all caffeine and alcohol, both powerful stimulants that can raise blood pressure in sensitive people. The food is low sodium and high potassium; and most important, circulation improves shortly after starting a low-fat diet. Most of the patients at our clinic are off their medication in just one day and their blood pressure is lower than it was when they were on medication. The average drop is 6 mm Hg in the top number (systolic) and 3 mm Hg in the bottom number (diastolic). People initially with blood pressures greater than 150/90 show an even greater pressure reduction. The average drop is 20 mm Hg in the top number and 11 mm Hg in the bottom number. In most cases their medications were stopped on day one of our program—unless they were on B-blockers or large amounts of medications.

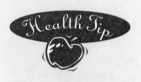

Health Tip

Anxiety over seeing your doctor can raise your blood pressure. People with high blood pressure should monitor it at home for the most accurate readings, and take your findings to your doctor. This way you'll avoid blood pressure pills to treat the fear of your doctor.

Cilantro Soup

Servings: 6
Preparation Time:
10 minutes
Cooking Time:
20 minutes

6 cups vegetable broth
6 cups frozen chopped hash
brown potatoes
1 cup cilantro leaves

1 teaspoon minced fresh garlic
1 teaspoon Tabasco sauce
¼ cup lemon juice

Place the broth and potatoes in a large saucepan. Bring to a boil. Cook over medium heat for 15 minutes. Remove from heat. Add the cilantro, garlic, and Tabasco sauce. Puree in batches in a blender or food processor. Return to the pan and heat through, about 5 minutes. Stir in the lemon juice just before serving.

Recipe Hint: *If you are a cilantro lover, this soup could well become one of your favorites. If you don't like cilantro, try this with parsley.*

Speedy Gazpacho

Servings: 6 to 8
Preparation Time:
10 minutes
Chilling Time:
2 hours

1 cucumber
1 green bell pepper
1 stalk celery

2 green onions
1 32-ounce jar spicy tomato juice
several dashes of Tabasco sauce

Chop all the vegetables in large chunks. Using a blender, process the vegetables in batches in the tomato juice. Add the Tabasco sauce, mix well, and place in a large covered jar or pitcher. Refrigerate at least 2 hours to blend the flavors.

Recipe Hint: *We make this very often during the summer for a fast meal or a snack. Just pour it into a mug and drink it on the road. It is delicious and very refreshing.*

Quick Kasba Curry Soup

⅓ cup water
1 onion, chopped
1 stalk celery, chopped

4 cups vegetable broth
3 cups cooked brown rice
1 to 2 teaspoons curry powder

Servings: 4
Preparation Time:
5 minutes
(need cooked rice)
Cooking Time:
35 minutes

Place the water, onion, and celery in a saucepan. Cook, stirring occasionally, for 5 minutes. Add the remaining ingredients. Cook over low heat for 30 minutes longer.

Recipe Hint: *If you're not sure how spicy you like your soup, start with 1 teaspoon of curry powder and then add more if you really love curry.*

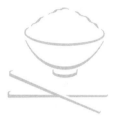

Creamy Pumpkin Soup

¼ cup water
1 small onion, chopped
4 cups vegetable broth
1 16-ounce can solid-pack
  pumpkin

½ cup unsweetened applesauce
2 teaspoons curry powder
several dashes of Tabasco
  sauce
½ cup soy or rice milk

Servings: 6
Preparation Time:
5 minutes
Cooking Time:
10 minutes

Place the water and onion in a medium saucepan. Cook, stirring occasionally, for 5 minutes, until the onion is soft. Add the broth, pumpkin, and applesauce. Stir to combine. Add the seasonings. Cook over low heat, stirring occasionally, for 10 minutes. Stir in the milk just before serving.

Recipe Hint: *This would be very attractive served in a small baked pumpkin. Cut the top off a pumpkin. Clean out the seeds and strings as you would for a Halloween jack-o'-lantern. Replace the top. Place the pumpkin in a pan with ½ inch of water. Bake at 350 degrees for 30 minutes.*

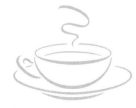

Chinese Noodle Soup

Servings: 4
Preparation Time:
5 minutes
Cooking Time:
15 minutes

6 cups vegetable broth
2 tablespoons soy sauce
½ teaspoon minced garlic
½ teaspoon minced fresh
gingerroot

5 ounces Chinese noodles
4 to 5 green onions, sliced into
½-inch pieces

Place the broth, soy sauce, garlic, and ginger in a saucepan. Bring to a boil and add the remaining ingredients. Reduce heat and simmer for 10 minutes, stirring frequently to break apart the noodles.

Recipe Hint: *To add a bit more character to this soup, we add a few canned straw mushrooms, some canned baby corn, and a handful or two of fresh chopped spinach. The brand of noodles that we use is China Bowl Select, made by China Bowl Trading Co. You can buy them in natural food stores.*

Creamy Vege Soup

Servings: 4 to 6
Preparation Time:
10 minutes
Cooking Time:
15 minutes

2½ cups water
1 head cauliflower, cut into large
pieces
1 small onion, coarsely chopped
1 teaspoon minced fresh garlic
1 cup frozen chopped hash
brown potatoes

½ cup baby carrots
1 stalk celery, coarsely
chopped
¼ cup soy sauce
½ cup cashews
¾ teaspoon cardamom

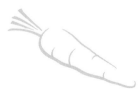

Combine all ingredients in a large soup pot. Bring to a boil, cover, and cook over medium heat for 15 minutes, or until all the vegetables are tender. Blend in batches in a food processor or blender and serve hot, garnished with thinly sliced green onions, if desired.

WHICH FOOD STORE?

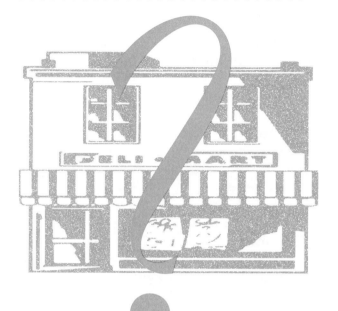

$\mathcal{S}$hould you shop in a health food store, a natural food store, or a supermarket? The typical health food store often emphasizes high-profit vitamins and supplements rather than wholesome foods. Natural food stores stock wholesome packaged foods and fresh fruits and vegetables. Supermarkets sell what every American shopper wants regardless of the nutritional value. The distinction between natural food stores and supermarkets is diminishing. Supermarkets are catering to the customers' demands for healthier foods. Natural food stores have expanded to the size of supermarkets and sell everything from dog food to toilet paper (recycled, of course). The increased volume of sales has brought the cost of healthy foods down in both kinds of stores.

If you live near a large natural food store, this is where you will likely choose to shop. If not, then you should buy most of your whole grains, fruits, and vegetables at the supermarket, and your specialty needs, such as low-fat soy cheese, tofu, and packaged whole foods, at the health food store. Mail-order companies also sell almost everything you need at reasonable prices (see *The New McDougall Cookbook*).

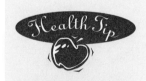

Buy fresh. Spoilage allows molds to grow on cereals and nuts which can produce powerful cancer-causing, liver-damaging chemicals, called aflatoxins. Spoiled potatoes contain intestine-distressing solanine toxins.

Greeny Beany Soup

Servings: 6
Preparation Time:
15 minutes
Cooking Time:
25 minutes

5 cups vegetable broth
3 leeks, white part only, thinly
    sliced
1 large red potato, scrubbed and
    chopped
1 teaspoon dried basil
1 teaspoon dried oregano
several generous twists of freshly
    ground black pepper

½ cup orzo
1 15-ounce can white beans,
    drained and rinsed
2 small zucchini, cut in half
    lengthwise, then sliced
2 to 3 cups packed chopped fresh
    spinach
several dashes of Tabasco
    sauce

Pour 1 cup of the broth into a large pot. Add the leeks. Cook, stirring occasionally, for 3 minutes. Add the remaining 4 cups broth, the
potato, basil, oregano and pepper. Cover and cook for 5 minutes.
Add the orzo and continue to cook for 5 more minutes, stirring occasionally. Add the beans and zucchini and continue to cook for
10 more minutes. Stir in the spinach and Tabasco. Cook until the
spinach has wilted, about 2 minutes.

Recipe Hint: *Buy triple-washed spinach in bags. Remove the*
stems and stack the leaves in piles. Cut down the center length-
wise, then slice crosswise. Orzo is a small rice-shaped pasta
that cooks very quickly. It is sold in supermarkets and natural
food stores.

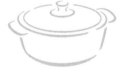

Black-Eyed Pea and Spinach Soup

1 10-ounce package frozen
   black-eyed peas
2½ cups vegetable broth
1 14.5-ounce can chopped
   tomatoes

1 8-ounce can tomato
   sauce
1 cup salsa
1 10-ounce package frozen
   chopped spinach

Place the peas and vegetable broth in a medium saucepan. Bring to a boil, cover, and cook over low heat for 15 minutes. Add the remaining ingredients and cook, stirring occasionally, until the spinach has thawed and the soup is heated through, about 5 minutes.

Onion Soup

5 cups vegetable broth
3 large onions, cut in half
   lengthwise and then sliced
¼ cup sherry
2 tablespoons Worcestershire sauce
1 tablespoon soy sauce

1 teaspoon dried minced onion
½ teaspoon minced fresh garlic
½ teaspoon onion powder
¼ teaspoon ground thyme
several twists of freshly ground
   black pepper

Place ½ cup of the broth in a large soup pot. Add the onions. Cook over medium heat, stirring frequently, for 10 minutes. Add the remaining ingredients, bring to a boil, cover, and cook for 20 minutes.

Recipe Hint: Serve with a hearty loaf of bread to dunk in the flavorful broth. Or make some whole wheat croutons to float in the soup. Preheat the oven to 350 degrees. Cut slices of whole wheat bread into cubes. Place on a baking sheet and toast for 5 to 10 minutes. Or use a toaster oven if you have one. Place the cubes in the tray and toast for a few minutes.

Servings: 6
Preparation Time: 5 minutes
Cooking Time: 20 minutes

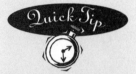

Have your freezer stocked with frozen staples like artichoke hearts, baby lima beans, black-eyed peas, cauliflower, chopped broccoli, corn kernels, cooked pureed winter squash, chopped spinach, and hash brown potatoes. Boil into delicious side dishes. Add to soups and stews for color, flavor, texture, and body.

Servings: 4
Preparation Time: 10 minutes
Cooking Time: 30 minutes

POTS AND PANS

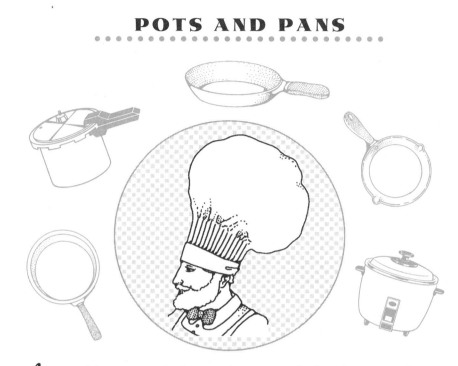

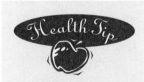
Acceptable materials for cookware include glass, stainless steel, iron, nonstick-coated pans and bake ware (such as Dupont's Silverstone, Teflon, or Farberware Millennium), silicone-coated bake ware (such as Baker's Secret), and porcelain. Nonstick cookware makes it easy to avoid fats and oil. We recommend that you avoid using aluminum cookware because of an association with Alzheimer's disease. Buy one each of the following cookware, unless otherwise specified:

2-quart saucepan
3-quart saucepan
4-quart saucepan
6-quart stockpot
8-quart steamer/pasta cooker
12-quart stockpot
griddle
large frying pan
electric wok
9¼ × 5¼ loaf pan

8 × 8 × 2 square baking pan
9 × 13 × 2 oblong baking pan
baking trays (2)
2-quart covered casserole dish
3-quart covered casserole dish
6-quart square covered casserole dish
9 × 13 oblong uncovered baking dishes (2)
7½ × 11¾ oblong uncovered baking dish
muffin tin
rice cooker

Cream of Vegetable Soup

5 cups vegetable broth
1 onion, cut in chunks
3 cups vegetables, cut in chunks

½ cup rolled oats
seasonings of your choice
    (see hint)

Servings: 4
Preparation Time:
10 minutes
Cooking Time:
30 minutes

Combine all ingredients in a medium soup pot, bring to a boil, and simmer for 30 minutes. Puree in batches in a food processor or blender. Serve at once.

Recipe Hint: *For seasoning try one of the following: 1 teaspoon dill weed; ½ teaspoon thyme and ½ teaspoon marjoram; 1 teaspoon ground cumin; ½ teaspoon basil and ¼ teaspoon oregano.*

Cut the vegetables any old way because they all get pureed at the end. Use one kind of vegetable only or a combination of what you have on hand—cauliflower, broccoli, carrots, celery, spinach, etc.

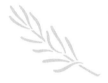

Potato Chowder

Servings: 4 to 6
Preparation Time:
10 minutes
Cooking Time:
25 minutes

3½ cups vegetable broth
6 cups frozen chopped hash
    brown potatoes
1 onion, chopped
2 small stalks celery, chopped
1 small leek, sliced

½ teaspoon salt (optional)
⅛ teaspoon white pepper
2 cups soy or rice milk
1 to 2 tablespoons parsley flakes
1 to 2 tablespoons dried chives
dash of liquid smoke

Place the broth, potatoes, onion, celery, and leek in a large pot. Bring to a boil. Cover, reduce heat, and cook for 20 minutes. Remove 3 cups from the pot and place in a blender jar. Process until smooth and then return to the pot. Add the remaining ingredients. Cook until heated through, about 5 minutes.

Vegetable broth in a can, vegetable bouillon cubes, or vegetable bouillon powder is used as a base for soups and gravies. Try broth for sautéing.

Mexi Corn Chowder

Servings: 4
Preparation Time:
10 minutes
Cooking Time:
10 minutes

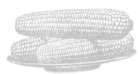

¼ cup water
1 cup chopped green onions
3 cups frozen corn kernels, thawed
2 cups soy or rice milk

2 tablespoons chopped pimiento
2 tablespoons chopped canned green chilies
dash or two of Tabasco sauce
chopped cilantro for garnish

Place the water and onions in a saucepan. Cook, stirring frequently, for 3 minutes. Add the corn and milk. Bring to a boil, reduce heat, and simmer for 5 minutes. Remove 1 cup to a blender jar and process until smooth. Return to the pan. Add the remaining ingredients, except the cilantro, and heat through, about 2 minutes. Garnish with the cilantro before serving.

Chunky Vegetable Chowder

Servings: 4
Preparation Time:
15 minutes
Cooking Time:
12 minutes

2 cups red potatoes, cut into chunks
2½ cups vegetable broth
½ cup chopped onion
½ cup chopped green bell pepper
½ cup chopped red bell pepper

½ cup chopped yellow or orange bell pepper
¼ cup unbleached white flour
3 cups soy or rice milk
1 tablespoon soy sauce
2 teaspoons chopped fresh basil
¼ teaspoon ground white pepper

Place the potatoes and 2 cups of the broth in a saucepan. Bring to a boil, reduce heat, cover, and cook for 10 minutes. Set aside. Do not drain.

Meanwhile, place the remaining ½ cup vegetable broth in another saucepan. Add the onion and bell peppers. Cook, stirring occasionally, for 6 minutes. Stir in the flour. Add the remaining ingredients and cook, stirring frequently, until thickened. Add the cooked potatoes and broth. Heat through and serve.

Corn Chowder

3 cups vegetable broth
1 onion, chopped
2 cups frozen chopped hash
  brown potatoes
2 cups frozen corn kernels
1 teaspoon Worcestershire sauce
½ teaspoon thyme

¼ teaspoon dry mustard
¼ teaspoon paprika
¼ teaspoon marjoram
2 tablespoons diced pimiento
½ cup soy or rice milk
freshly ground black pepper to
  taste

Place the broth, onion, potatoes, and corn in a medium soup pot. Bring to a boil, add the seasonings, cover, and simmer for 25 minutes. Remove 2 cups of the soup and place in a blender. Blend until smooth. Return to the pot. Add the pimiento and milk. Season with the pepper. Cook for an additional 5 minutes.

Summer Vegetable Bisque

½ cup water
1 onion, chopped
½ teaspoon minced fresh garlic
1 red or green bell pepper,
  chopped
3 tablespoons unbleached flour
3 cups vegetable broth
2 zucchini, diced

2 cups frozen corn kernels
2 cups chopped fresh tomatoes
1 tablespoon soy sauce
¾ teaspoon ground cumin
¾ teaspoon dill weed
⅛ teaspoon white pepper
1½ cups soy or rice milk

Place the water in a large soup pot. Add the onion, garlic, and bell pepper. Cook, stirring frequently, for 3 to 4 minutes. Mix in the flour. Add the broth, zucchini, corn, tomatoes, and seasonings. Cover, bring to a boil, reduce heat, and simmer for 10 minutes. Stir in the milk. Heat through and serve.

Servings: 4
Preparation Time:
10 minutes
Cooking Time:
30 minutes

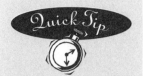

As frozen, partially pre-cooked hash brown potatoes cook, they soften and break apart, adding extra body to soups and stews.

Servings: 6
Preparation Time:
15 minutes
Cooking Time:
14 minutes

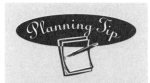

Make meals easier and more fun by involving friends and family in the meal preparations. This idea can also work outside the home. Ask coworkers, friends, and family who live apart to make large enough dishes to share.

Creamy Green Onion Soup

Servings: 6 to 8
Preparation Time:
15 minutes
Cooking Time:
25 minutes

6 cups water
4 cups frozen chopped hash
   brown potatoes
1½ cups celery
3 cups chopped green onions
3 teaspoons vegetable broth
   seasoning mix

1 tablespoon soy sauce
1 tablespoon parsley flakes
1 teaspoon dill weed
1 teaspoon paprika
several twists of freshly ground
   black pepper
several dashes of Tabasco sauce

Place the water in a large soup pot. Add the potatoes and celery. Bring to a boil. Add 2½ cups of the green onions to the pot. Add the seasonings and cook over medium heat for 20 minutes. Puree the soup in batches in a blender. Return to the pot, add the remaining ½ cup of green onions, and cook for an additional 5 minutes.

> **Recipe Hint:** *To turn this into a curried soup, add 1 teaspoon of curry powder instead of the paprika.*

Servings: 8
Preparation Time:
10 minutes
Cooking Time:
34 minutes

Chilly Kale Soup

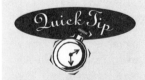

Use a food processor to shred onions, carrots, celery, peppers, mushrooms, zucchini, kale, parsley, and cilantro into bite-size pieces in seconds.

8 cups vegetable broth
1 onion, chopped
1 teaspoon minced fresh garlic
¾ cup red lentils
1 14.5-ounce can chopped
   tomatoes
1 tablespoon chili powder

½ teaspoon ground cumin
2 bay leaves
4 cups chopped fresh kale
2 cups frozen chopped hash
   brown potatoes
1 cup frozen corn kernels
2 tablespoons soy sauce

Place ⅓ cup of the vegetable broth in a large soup pan. Add the onion and garlic. Cook, stirring frequently, for 4 minutes. Add the remaining broth, lentils, tomatoes, chili powder, cumin, and bay leaves. Cover, bring to a boil, reduce heat, and cook for 15 minutes. Add the remaining ingredients and cook for 15 minutes longer.

READING LABELS

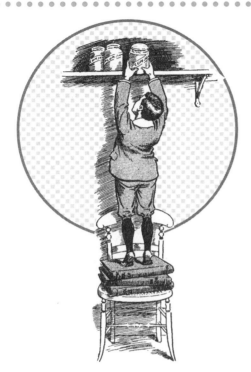

$\mathcal{Y}$ou must know how to read labels in order to wisely buy packaged goods. Ingredients are listed in descending order based on their weight. Manufacturers can slide an unhealthy ingredient toward the bottom of the list by using a variety of names to describe it. For example, sugars can be listed individually as sucrose, fructose, dextrose, maltose, and multidextran. If they were all grouped together as simple sugar then this ingredient would be first on the list.

Manufacturers use unfamiliar names to disguise harmful ingredients. Fats and oils are hidden by calling them monoglycerides and diglycerides (you might recognize triglyceride as a name for fats) or lecithin, which is a fat made from soybeans. Dairy products are concealed as whey, casein, and lactose.

Buy products that have no oils or animals products and few additives. Avoid overrefined and overprocessed foods. If you can't pronounce an ingredient on the package, or have never heard of it, you probably shouldn't be eating it.

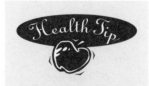

By government regulation, "fat-free" means that a single serving contains less than ½ gram of fat. The claim fat-free can be accomplished by making the serving size small enough to fit the rules, yet the ingredient list contains fats and oils.

Succotash Soup

Servings: 6 to 8
Preparation Time:
15 minutes
Cooking Time:
25 minutes

½ cup water
1 onion, chopped
1 stalk celery, chopped
2 cups vegetable broth
1 14.5-ounce can chopped
   tomatoes
1 red bell pepper, chopped
2 cups frozen chopped hash
   brown potatoes

1 cup frozen lima beans
1 tablespoon parsley flakes
1 teaspoon Dijon–style
   mustard
1 teaspoon honey
several twists of freshly ground
   black pepper
2 cups frozen corn kernels
2½ cups soy or rice milk

Place the water in a large pot. Add the onion and celery. Cook, stirring frequently, for 3 to 4 minutes. Add the remaining ingredients, except for the corn and milk. Bring to a boil, reduce heat, cover, and simmer for 15 minutes. Add the corn and milk and cook for an additional 5 minutes. Remove 1 to 2 cups of the soup from the pot. Place in a blender jar and process until smooth. Return to the pot and mix well.

Cooking Tip

To thicken soups or stews, remove about one-quarter from the pot, blend in a food processor or blender until smooth, then return to the pot and stir.

Mexican Tomato-Potato Soup

Servings: 6
Preparation Time:
10 minutes
Cooking Time:
25 minutes

2 onions, chopped
2 teaspoons minced fresh garlic
4 cups vegetable broth
1 15-ounce can chopped
   tomatoes
3 cups frozen chopped hash
   brown potatoes

2 tablespoons chopped canned
   green chilies
1 teaspoon dried oregano
freshly ground black pepper to
   taste
¼ cup chopped cilantro
1 tablespoon lime juice

Place the onions and garlic in a sauce pot with ½ cup of the vegetable broth. Cook, stirring occasionally, for 4 minutes. Add the remaining broth, tomatoes, potatoes, chilies, oregano, and pepper. Bring to a boil, reduce heat, and simmer for 20 minutes. Stir in the cilantro and lime juice just before serving.

Cream of Mushroom Soup

1 onion, chopped
½ pound fresh button
　mushrooms, chopped
8 fresh shiitake mushrooms,
　chopped
10 fresh oyster mushrooms,
　chopped

½ cup white wine
5 cups vegetable broth
2 cups frozen chopped hash
　brown potatoes
1 tablespoon parsley flakes
¼ teaspoon nutmeg
2½ cups soy milk

Servings: 6
Preparation Time:
15 minutes
Cooking Time:
30 minutes

Place the onion and mushrooms in a large pot with the wine. Cook, stirring frequently, for 5 minutes. Add the broth, potatoes, parsley, and nutmeg. Cover and cook over low heat for 20 minutes. Add the soy milk and cook for an additional 5 minutes.

Process in batches in a food processor or blender. Return to the pot and heat through.

Recipe Hint: *Serve this delicious, thick, creamy mushroom soup with thick slices of fresh bread to dunk.*

GENERAL DISEASE CATEGORIES

chronic illness
"Multiple Injury"

acute illness
"Single Injury"

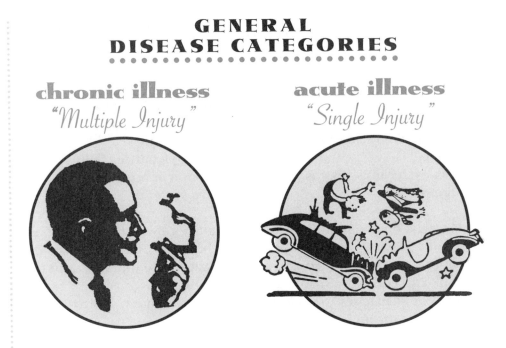

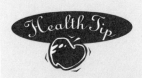

We all know good health is supported by clean water and air, moderate exercise, and adequate rest. Confusion exists over the right diet. People who avoid diseases common to Americans eat a mostly vegetarian diet.

*M*odern medicine succeeds with problems that can be classified as *acute illnesses*. These are *single* assaults on the body, such as a laceration caused by a knife blade, a bone broken by a fall, or an infection of the bladder by a bacteria. When a doctor sutures the laceration, straightens the bone, or administers an antibiotic he or she tilts the balance in favor of the patient's recovery.

Most illnesses people suffer from are classified as *chronic illnesses*. These include obesity, diabetes, hypertension, heart disease, cancer, indigestion, and constipation. Chronic illness is a result of repeated injuries. For example, coughing, wheezing, and shortness of breath may be due to lung disease caused by cigarette smoking, a common behavior. "Acute care" solutions like cough syrups and pills to control wheezing do not solve the problem. The solution is to stop the repeated injury. Coughing and wheezing disappear within a week after you stop smoking as your body heals from the smoke-induced damage. To solve other chronic illnesses we must find the source of repeated injury.

Curried Swiss Chard Soup

⅓ cup water
2 leeks, thinly sliced
1¾ cups vegetable broth
1 14.5-ounce can chopped
   tomatoes
1 15-ounce can white beans,
   drained and rinsed

2 teaspoons curry powder
2 teaspoons minced fresh
   gingerroot
1 teaspoon sugar
4 cups finely chopped Swiss
   chard

Servings: 4
Preparation Time:
15 minutes
Cooking Time:
18 minutes

Place the water in a large soup pot. Add the leeks and cook, stirring frequently, for 2 minutes. Add the remaining ingredients, except for the Swiss chard. Bring to a boil, cover, reduce heat, and simmer for 15 minutes. Add the Swiss chard, stir, and cook until wilted, about 1 minute. Serve at once.

Recipe Hint: *Chop the Swiss chard in a food processor to save time. Other green leafy vegetables may be substituted for the Swiss chard, such as mustard greens, kale, or escarole.*

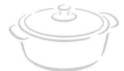

Fast Minestrone

Servings: 6
Preparation Time:
10 minutes
Cooking Time:
30 minutes

3 cups vegetable broth
1 14.5-ounce can Italian-style
    stewed tomatoes
½ cup uncooked small pasta
1 15-ounce can kidney beans,
    drained and rinsed
1 15-ounce can cannellini beans,
    drained and rinsed

1 16-ounce package frozen
    Italian-style mixed
    vegetables
2 teaspoons parsley flakes
½ teaspoon basil
½ teaspoon marjoram
freshly ground black pepper to
    taste

Combine all ingredients in a large sauce pot. Bring to a boil, reduce heat, cover, and simmer for 30 minutes.

Recipe Hint: *Serve hot with a loaf of fresh bread for a delicious, hearty meal. Our original minestrone recipe took a lot more time to prepare and cook, but by using canned beans, seasoned canned tomatoes, and frozen precut vegetables this delicious soup can be on the table in a half hour.*

Mexi Soup

1 onion, chopped
⅓ cup water
1 28-ounce can crushed tomatoes
1 15-ounce can kidney beans,
    undrained
1 15-ounce can garbanzo beans,
    undrained

1 16-ounce can creamed corn
1 cup vegetable broth
1 8-ounce can tomato sauce
1 tablespoon taco seasoning
several dashes of Tabasco
    sauce

Servings: 6
Preparation Time:
5 minutes
Cooking Time:
30 minutes

Place the onion and water in a medium soup pot. Cook, stirring occasionally, for 4 minutes. Add the remaining ingredients, bring to a boil, cover, and simmer for 25 minutes.

Recipe Hint: *We use Taco Dust seasoning by Cajun Dust of Phoenix, Arizona. Other taco seasonings will also work in this recipe. This spicy, thick soup is hearty enough for a filling dinner when served with a loaf of bread.*

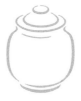

Mexican Black Bean Tortilla Soup

2 15-ounce cans black beans
1 15-ounce can fat-free vegetable
    soup
1½ cups water
1 11-ounce can corn

1 15-ounce can chopped
    tomatoes
½ cup salsa
2 cups baked fat-free tortilla
    chips

Servings: 4
Preparation Time:
5 minutes
Cooking Time:
20 minutes

Combine all ingredients, except the chips, in a saucepan. Simmer over low heat for 20 minutes. Break up the chips slightly and place ½ cup in the bottom of a soup bowl. Ladle the soup over the chips and let rest for a minute or two to soften the chips. Repeat with the remaining chips and soup.

Cajun Gumbo

Servings: 6 to 8
Preparation Time:
10 minutes
Cooking Time:
30 minutes

4 cups vegetable broth
1 onion, chopped
1 green bell pepper, chopped
1 stalk celery, chopped
1 teaspoon minced fresh garlic
1 15-ounce can Cajun-style
  stewed tomatoes

1½ cups frozen lima beans
1½ cups frozen sliced okra
1 cup frozen corn kernels
1 teaspoon paprika
½ teaspoon gumbo filé (optional)
dash of cayenne pepper
several dashes of Tabasco sauce

Place ½ cup of the broth in a large sauce pot. Add the onion, bell pepper, celery, and garlic. Cook, stirring occasionally, for 5 minutes. Add the remaining ingredients. Bring to a boil, reduce heat, cover, and simmer for 25 minutes.

Recipe Hint: Gumbo filé is an ingredient often used in Southern cooking. It is made from sassafras leaves. It can be found in most supermarkets in the spice section.

FOUR OR MORE
FEASTS A DAY!

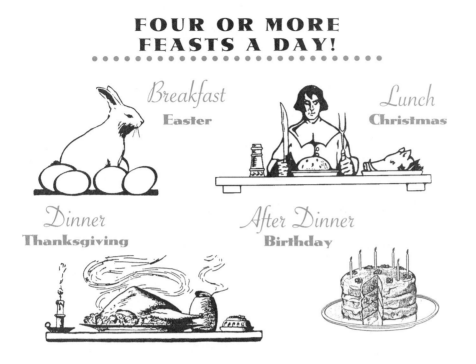

Breakfast
Easter

Lunch
Christmas

Dinner
Thanksgiving

After Dinner
Birthday

Throughout history most people have lived on diets based on starches such as rice in Asia, pasta in southern Europe, and corn and beans in South America. But all societies have celebrations, and on these days people do extraordinary things: They take the day off from work, dance in the streets, watch athletic games, and eat rich foods. In the past, a few rich people—royalty and fellow aristocrats—decided to make every day a special occasion. The results of all that feasting are obvious from literature and art: Wealthy people are pictured sitting uncomfortably with their gout-inflicted feet propped on a stool.

Today, many Americans can afford to eat like royalty. For breakfast we have eggs, an Easter tradition. At lunch and dinner we feast on Thanksgiving and Christmas favorites—turkeys and hams, creamy sauces and thick gravies, and butter-soaked breads and vegetables. And we top it all off with cake and ice cream. The consequences of this diet are the same today as they were in the past. Eating foods loaded with fat, cholesterol, sugar, and salt, and deficient in vitamins, minerals, and dietary fiber, causes repeated injury to the body. The solution is to make feasts special again and to eat foods designed for healthy human beings every day.

Health Tip

Human beings are designed to survive. We live on two packages of cigarettes, a half bottle of whiskey, and the wrong fuel, daily, and survive. Imagine the consequences of taking excellent care of ourselves.

Miso Vegetable Broth

Servings: 2
Preparation Time:
10 minutes
Cooking Time:
10 minutes

3½ cups vegetable broth
1 bunch green onions, chopped
1 carrot, thinly sliced
1 stalk celery, sliced
½ cup uncooked vegetable rotelli
½ cup sliced fresh mushrooms

½ cup frozen peas
½ cup frozen corn kernels
1½ tablespoons light miso
½ tablespoon chopped cilantro or
    parsley

Place the broth in a saucepan. Add the green onions, carrot, celery, and pasta. Bring to a boil, cover, reduce heat, and simmer for 5 minutes. Add the mushrooms, peas, and corn. Continue to cook for 5 minutes. Remove a small amount of broth to a bowl. Stir in the miso and mix well. Add to the soup along with the cilantro. Mix well and serve.

Recipe Hint: This is a good way to use up some of the vegetables in your refrigerator and freezer. Keep the pieces small or thin so that they cook quickly. You can also use other pastas.

Creamy Carrot Soup

Servings: 6
Preparation Time:
15 minutes
Cooking Time:
20 minutes

5 cups vegetable broth
1 pound carrots, chopped
2 cups sliced leeks
2 cups frozen chopped hash
    brown potatoes

½ teaspoon minced fresh
    garlic
¼ teaspoon white pepper
¼ teaspoon dill weed

Combine all ingredients in a pot. Bring to a boil, reduce heat, cover, and cook for 20 minutes. Puree the soup in batches in a blender. Return to the pan and heat through. Serve warm or cold.

Recipe Hint: Turn this into a curried carrot soup by adding 2 teaspoons curry powder, 2 teaspoons minced fresh gingerroot, and 1 teaspoon ground coriander.

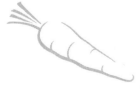

Chili Tortilla Soup

⅓ cup water
1 leek, thinly sliced
1 cup chopped celery
½ teaspoon minced fresh garlic
1¾ cups vegetable broth
1 7-ounce can chopped green
    chilies
2 cups soy or rice milk

½ teaspoon ground cumin
dash or two of Tabasco sauce
1 tablespoon cornstarch mixed in
    ¼ cup cold water
1 cup baked fat-free tortilla
    chips, broken into pieces
chopped cilantro for garnish

Servings: 4
Preparation Time:
10 minutes
Cooking Time:
10 minutes

Place the water in a large pot with the leek, celery, and garlic. Cook, stirring occasionally, for 3 to 4 minutes, until softened. Add the broth, chilies, milk, cumin, and Tabasco. Cook over low heat, stirring occasionally, for 5 minutes. Stir in the cornstarch mixture and cook and stir until slightly thickened. Place ¼ cup of the chips into each of 4 bowls and ladle the soup over the chips. Garnish with the cilantro.

A MUSCLE IS A MUSCLE IS A MUSCLE

Cholesterol in Meats (mg/3.5 ounces)

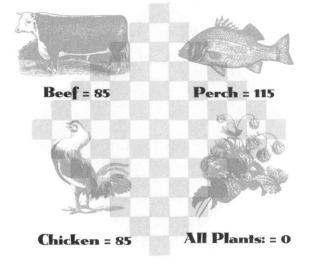

Beef = 85　　　**Perch = 115**

Chicken = 85　　　**All Plants: = 0**

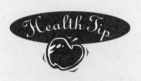

Red meat, poultry, and fish are all high-protein and/or high-fat; contain no carbohydrate or dietary fiber; contain high levels of environmental contaminants and cholesterol; are deficient in vitamin C and calcium; and often contain infectious organisms. Minimize risk ... eat less red and white meat.

*J*ohn sees patients every week who tell him that they went to the doctor for treatment of elevated cholesterol and were told to switch from red meat (beef and pork) to white meat (chicken and fish). Some time later their cholesterol tests were repeated and the level was still high. These patients believe they have a "genetic disease," but the truth is they have an "information disease." The cholesterol content of various muscles is essentially the same. Switching among them for your meals will leave you with the same health problems. Four scientific experiments have been done where people are switched from red meat to white meat and all four found the subjects' cholesterol levels remained the same after the change. A muscle is a muscle is a muscle, whether it wiggles a tail, flaps a wing, moves a limb, or closes a shell.

Black Bean Soup

¼ cup water
1 small onion, chopped
½ teaspoon minced garlic
3 15-ounce cans black beans
1½ cups water
1 8-ounce can tomato sauce
½ teaspoon ground cumin

½ teaspoon chili powder
1 teaspoon lemon juice
dash or two of Tabasco sauce
freshly ground black pepper to
taste
chopped cilantro and green
onions for garnish (optional)

Servings: 4 to 6
Preparation Time:
10 minutes
Cooking Time:
20 minutes

Place the ¼ cup water in a large saucepan with the onion and garlic. Cook and stir over medium-high heat until the onion softens slightly, about 3 minutes. Add the remaining ingredients, except the garnish. Bring to a boil, cover, reduce heat, and cook for 15 minutes. Garnish with cilantro and green onions, if desired.

Recipe Hint: For a thicker soup, remove some of the beans to a separate bowl and mash before returning to the pan. This makes the soup taste just as rich as if it had cooked all day.

Hearty White Bean Soup

½ cup water
1 onion, chopped
2 carrots, sliced
1 stalk celery, sliced
1½ cups shredded cabbage
1 teaspoon minced fresh garlic
2 15-ounce cans white beans,
drained and rinsed

4 cups vegetable broth
2 cups frozen chopped hash
brown potatoes
1 bay leaf
1 tablespoon soy sauce
1 tablespoon parsley flakes
several twists of freshly ground
black pepper

Servings: 8
Preparation Time:
15 minutes
Cooking Time:
30 minutes

Place the water in a large pot. Add the onion, carrots, celery, cabbage, and garlic. Cook, stirring frequently, for 10 minutes. Add the remaining ingredients, bring to a boil, cover, reduce heat, and simmer for 20 minutes. Remove the bay leaf before serving.

Shredded cabbage is available in bags in the supermarket. It is washed and ready to use.

Italian Four Bean Soup

Servings: 8
Preparation Time:
10 minutes
Cooking Time:
25 minutes

⅓ cup water
1 onion, chopped
½ teaspoon minced garlic
1 bunch kale, chopped
3 cups vegetable broth
1 14.5-ounce can chopped
  tomatoes
1 15-ounce can kidney beans,
  drained and rinsed
1 15-ounce can garbanzo beans,
  drained and rinsed
1 15-ounce can red beans,
  drained and rinsed

1 15-ounce can white beans,
  drained and rinsed
1 teaspoon Italian seasoning
  mix
several twists of freshly ground
  black pepper
1 15-ounce can white beans,
  mashed
4 slices Yves Canadian Veggie
  Bacon, chopped
1 tablespoon soy parmesan
  cheese (optional)

Place the water, onion, and garlic in a large saucepan. Cook and stir for 3 minutes. Add the kale and cook and stir for 2 minutes. Add the broth, tomatoes, drained beans, Italian seasoning, and pepper. Bring to a boil, cover, and simmer for 10 minutes. Add the mashed beans, veggie bacon, and soy cheese, if desired. Cook for an additional 10 minutes.

Quick Tip

Place leftover bean and vegetable dishes in corn or wheat tortillas. Roll them up and place them in a baking dish. Freeze for later use. Pour enchilada, marinara, curry, or salsa sauce or a gravy over the frozen dish and heat in the microwave.

Ellen's Bean Soup

¼ cup water
1 onion, chopped
1 tablespoon chili powder
1 28-ounce can chopped
   tomatoes
1 15-ounce can black
   beans, drained and
   rinsed

1 15-ounce can pinto beans,
   drained and rinsed
1 15-ounce can kidney beans,
   drained and rinsed
1 4-ounce can diced green chilies
1 10-ounce can Ro-tel tomatoes
   and green chilies
4 cups vegetable broth

Servings: 8
Preparation Time:
5 minutes
Cooking Time:
35 minutes

Place the water in a large soup pot. Add the onion and chili powder. Cook, stirring occasionally, for 5 minutes. Add the remaining ingredients, bring to a boil, cover, reduce heat, and simmer for 30 minutes.

Recipe Hint: *Serve in a bowl with a loaf of fresh bread, or serve over grains, potatoes, toast, or muffins. This soup freezes well.*

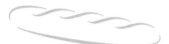

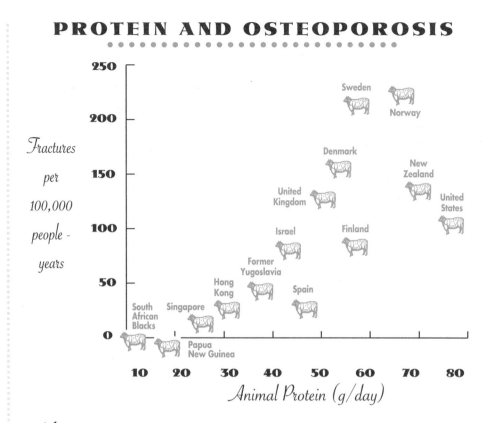

PROTEIN AND OSTEOPOROSIS

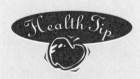

Health Tip

One to four percent of an adult's skeleton is lost every year while following the high protein American diet. Eventually the bones are so weak a cough breaks a rib and a normal step fractures a hip. Lack of exercise also weakens bones.

Hip fracture rates increase worldwide as animal protein intake in a population increases. In rural Africa and China, where people live on mostly vegetables, hip fractures are rare to nonexistent. In countries where meat, poultry, fish, and dairy products highlight the meals, hip fractures are common.

Proteins are made of amino *acids*. Because meat, poultry, fish, and eggs contain highly acidic amino acids, they provide an acid load to the body. Plant foods, on the other hand, provide an alkaline (base) load. The body protects its acid-base balance carefully so that biochemical reactions can occur properly. An acidic, animal food–based diet must be neutralized (buffered). The primary buffering system of the body is the bones. Bones dissolve to neutralize the acid. This is the first step to osteoporosis. Changes in kidney physiology cause the excretion of large amounts of calcium into the urine. This is the second step. The bones are weakened and the kidneys develop stones. Handfuls of calcium pills and gallons of milk will not make up for the loss. Lack of exercise, caffeine consumption, and early menopause also contribute in a small way to bone loss.

Bean and Corn Soup

½ cup minced onion
⅓ cup water
2 16-ounce cans nonfat
  refried beans, either pinto
  or black
1¾ cups vegetable broth
2 cups frozen corn kernels

½ cup mild or medium salsa
½ teaspoon ground cumin
several twists of freshly ground
  black pepper
dash or two of Tabasco sauce
Chopped fresh cilantro for
  garnish (optional)

Servings: 4
Preparation Time:
5 minutes
Cooking Time:
10 minutes

Place the onion and water in a saucepan. Cook, stirring occasionally, until the onion is soft, about 4 minutes. Add the beans and broth. Stir until well combined and souplike. Add the corn, salsa, cumin, and pepper. Cook, stirring occasionally, for 5 to 6 minutes, until heated through. Add the Tabasco sauce to taste. Garnish with the cilantro, if desired.

Recipe Hint: We like to make this with some of the new seasoned nonfat refried beans. Some of them are quite spicy, so you may want to cut down on the Tabasco sauce. Serve it in a bread bowl. Take a round loaf of bread and cut off the top. Hollow out the inside, leaving about ½ inch of the bread next to the crust. Serve the hot soup in the bread bowl. This soup is almost always a favorite with kids.

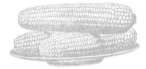

White Bean Soup

Servings: 4 to 6
Preparation Time:
10 minutes
Cooking Time:
19 minutes

⅓ cup water
1 onion, finely chopped
1 stalk celery, finely chopped
3 15-ounce cans white beans
2 cups vegetable broth

1 tablespoon soy sauce
1 bay leaf
½ teaspoon sage
½ teaspoon ground oregano
dash of liquid smoke

Place the water in a pot with the onion and celery. Cook, stirring frequently, until slightly softened, about 4 minutes. Add the remaining ingredients, bring to a boil, cover, reduce heat, and cook for 15 minutes. Remove the bay leaf before serving.

Recipe Hint: *For a thicker, creamy soup, remove 1 to 2 cups and place in a blender jar. Process until smooth and return to the pot. Our youngest son sometimes sprinkles curry powder on this soup and stirs it in before eating. We originally made it with dry white beans, but it took about 4 hours to cook. Now that canned and bottled beans are available, we can have this ready in a short time, and it's just as flavorful as the original. Chop the onions and celery in a food processor to save time. This is another favorite with kids.*

Spicy Lentil Soup

⅓ cup water
1 onion, sliced and separated
  into rings
1 stalk celery, chopped
1 carrot, chopped
1 teaspoon minced fresh
  garlic
6 cups vegetable broth
1 14.5-ounce can chopped
  tomatoes

1 cup dried red lentils
1 cup frozen chopped hash
  brown potatoes
2 tablespoons chopped canned
  green chilies
2 teaspoons chili powder
½ teaspoon ground oregano
½ cup uncooked whole wheat
  spaghetti, broken
¼ cup chopped cilantro

Servings: 6
Preparation Time:
10 minutes
Cooking Time:
35 minutes

Place the water in a large pot with the onion, celery, carrot, and garlic. Cook, stirring frequently, for 5 minutes. Add the broth, tomatoes, lentils, potatoes, green chilies, chili powder, and oregano. Bring to a boil, cover, reduce heat, and simmer for 20 minutes. Add the spaghetti and continue to cook for 10 more minutes. Stir in the cilantro and serve.

Tofu and Black Bean Stew

Servings: 2
Preparation Time:
5 minutes
Cooking Time:
30 minutes

1 10.5-ounce package firm lite silken tofu

1 15-ounce can black beans

1 14.5-ounce can Italian–style stewed tomatoes

1 4-ounce can sliced mushrooms, drained

Cube the tofu. Combine all ingredients in a medium saucepan. Cook over medium-low heat for 30 minutes, stirring occasionally.

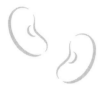

Recipe Hint: *Serve this with a green salad and French bread. You can use another style of stewed tomatoes, such as Cajun or Mexican.*

Speedy International Stew

Servings: 4
Preparation Time:
5 minutes
Cooking Time:
5 minutes

2 14.5-ounce cans stewed tomatoes (Italian, Mexican, or Cajun)

1 15-ounce can black beans, drained and rinsed

1 16-ounce can corn kernels, drained and rinsed

Place all ingredients in a medium saucepan and cook over medium heat for 5 minutes, stirring occasionally.

Recipe Hint: *This three-ingredient recipe is so simple you won't believe it can be so good. Serve with a loaf of fresh bread and a simple green salad for a hearty, quick meal.*

CALICUM AND OSTEOPOROSIS

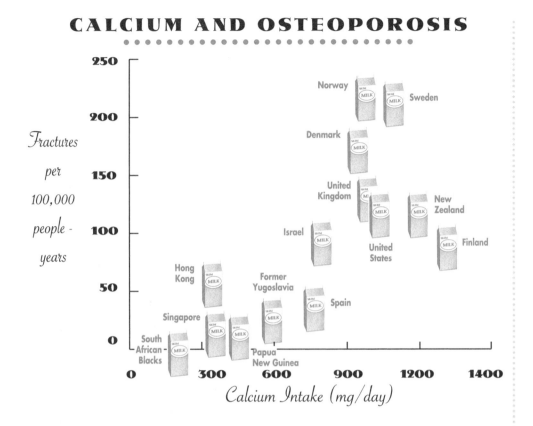

The more calcium consumed by a population the greater its incidence of osteoporosis. How can this be true if calcium is the main determinant of bone strength?

Calcium is a mineral found in the ground. Like all minerals it enters the food supply by dissolving in watery solutions and being absorbed by the roots of plants; it is then incorporated in the roots, stems, leaves, flowers, and fruits of plants. All animals obtain their minerals directly or indirectly (by eating other plant-eating animals) from plants. Calcium is important for bone health; however, all natural diets supply adequate amounts of calcium to meet human needs. Calcium deficiency of dietary origin is unknown in human beings. In other words, no one has ever developed a calcium deficiency because they ate a diet too low in calcium.

Osteoporosis is a dietary disease that is the direct result of eating too much meat, poultry, fish, and eggs. Because most of the food industry has a vested interest in selling us more protein and more calcium, they are unlikely to print the truth in their advertisements.

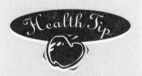

All unrefined plant foods are excellent sources of calcium—not just leafy green vegetables as taught by many nutrition experts. Minimum calcium requirements are as little as 200 milligrams daily. Worldwide, most populations consume 300-500 milligrams from plant foods and have strong skeletons.

Spicy Red Bean and Corn Stew

Servings: 6
Preparation Time:
10 minutes
Cooking Time:
20 minutes

¼ cup sherry
1 onion, chopped
1 stalk celery, chopped
1 green bell pepper, chopped
2 15-ounce cans red beans
2 cups frozen corn kernels

1 14.5-ounce can chopped tomatoes
1 teaspoon minced fresh garlic
2 teaspoons chili powder
2 teaspoons ground cumin
1 teaspoon ground oregano

Place the sherry, onion, celery, and bell pepper in a large pot. Cook over medium heat, stirring occasionally, for 5 minutes. Add the remaining ingredients. Bring to a boil, reduce heat, and simmer, uncovered, for 15 minutes. Serve over grains, bread or English muffins, or potatoes. Or serve in a bowl with some bread to dunk in the flavorful broth.

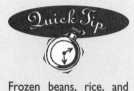

Quick Tip

Frozen beans, rice, and vegetables are quickly and easily thawed in 1 to 5 minutes by microwave.

Lima Bean Stew

Servings: 8
Preparation Time:
15 minutes
Cooking Time:
60 minutes

1 onion, chopped
1 red or green bell pepper, chopped
2 stalks celery, sliced
2 carrots, sliced
8 cups water
3 cups frozen lima beans
1 16-ounce can tomato sauce
¾ cup barley

¾ cup brown rice
2 tablespoons soy sauce
1 tablespoon parsley flakes
1 teaspoon dried basil
½ teaspoon paprika
½ teaspoon dried oregano
several twists of freshly ground black pepper

Combine all ingredients in a large soup pot. Bring to a boil, cover, reduce heat, and simmer for 60 minutes.

Recipe Hint: This may also be made in a slow cooker. Add all ingredients at once and cook on low for 4 to 6 hours. We have let this cook as long as 8 hours with no adverse results, except softer vegetables.

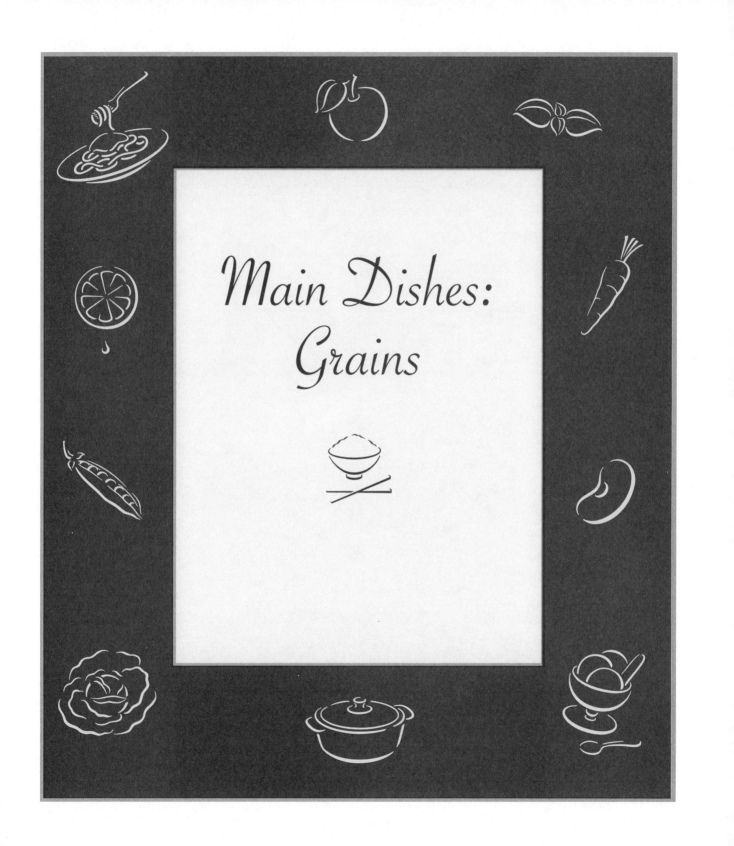

Main Dishes: Grains

Confetti Rice

½ cup water
1 red bell pepper, chopped
1 bunch green onions, chopped
1 cup frozen corn kernels
1 cup frozen baby lima beans
1 15-ounce can black beans,
    drained and rinsed

2 cups hot cooked brown rice
½ cup fat-free honey-mustard
    salad dressing
several twists of freshly ground
    black pepper

Servings: 4
Preparation Time:
10 minutes
(need cooked rice)
Cooking Time:
10 minutes

Place the water in a medium pot. Add the bell pepper, green onions, corn, and lima beans. Cook, stirring occasionally, for 10 minutes. Remove from heat and drain. Combine the vegetables, black beans, and rice. Add the dressing and toss to mix. Season with the pepper. Serve warm or cold.

Recipe Hint: *Use Success brand brown rice. It is precooked and ready to boil in a bag. It takes 10 minutes for hot, cooked rice. Substitute any of your favorite fat-free salad dressings for the honey-mustard dressing, if desired.*

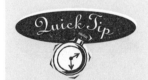

Flatten leftover rice or other grains or mashed potatoes into pancakes. Layer between plastic food wrap or parchment paper and freeze. Brown on a nonstick griddle or bake in the oven, serve with a gravy or sauce, or top with a cup of instant soup.

Quick Tip

Don't throw out that leftover rice. Put 1-cup portions in a plastic bag, or a bowl with a cover. Refrigerate or freeze for later use.

Spicy Spanish Rice

½ cup water
1 onion, chopped
1 teaspoon minced fresh garlic
1 green bell pepper, chopped
1 14.5-ounce can chopped
    tomatoes
1 tablespoon soy sauce
2 tablespoons chopped canned
    green chilies

4 cups cooked brown rice
2 tablespoons sliced black olives
    (optional)
1 teaspoon chili powder
½ teaspoon ground cumin
several dashes of Tabasco sauce
    (optional)

Place the water in a large pot. Add the onion, garlic, and green pepper. Cook, stirring frequently, for 5 minutes. Add the tomatoes, soy sauce, and chilies. Mix well. Stir in the rice and mix again. Add the remaining ingredients and cook for 15 minutes.

Quick Tip

There are many salsa flavors and degrees of hotness. Top burritos, tacos, tostados, salads, and stews with your favorite salsa to turn boring into blazing excitement. Salsa can also be added to soups and stews as they cook for more flavor.

Rice and
Beans in a Bowl

1 cup cooked brown rice
1 15-ounce can red or pinto
    beans, drained and rinsed
1 cup shredded lettuce
1 cup chopped tomato

1 green bell pepper,
    chopped
1 onion, chopped
¼ cup chopped cilantro
¾ cup salsa

Place the rice, beans, and half of each of the vegetables (not the salsa) in a microwave-safe bowl. Mix well, cover, and microwave on high for 3 minutes. Stir well and microwave for 2 more minutes. Stir in the remaining ingredients. Serve at once.

GRAINS—FAST & EASY

Grains

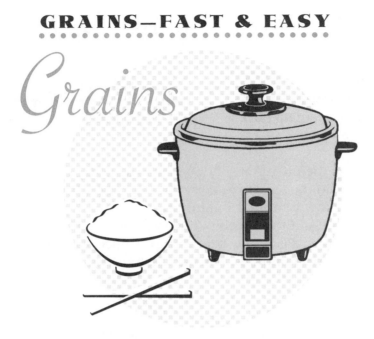

$\mathcal{M}$ost grains cook in boiling water in about forty-five minutes. Fast-cooking quinoa and bulgur take only fifteen minutes. For a fluffier texture let grains rest, uncovered, for fifteen minutes after cooking. Rice cookers cut cooking time and effort to a minimum, and they can cook every kind of grain to perfection. Buy a rice cooker with a nonstick coating on the liner surface. You can also buy one of the newer heavy plastic rice cooker/steamer models. Grains can also be cooked in a pressure cooker to save time. The best way to make grains convenient is to cook large amounts and then freeze leftovers in meal-size containers. Precooked white and brown rice sold as instant rice is quick and easy. Instant oatmeal is a thin slice of oats that cooks up faster. Instant grain breakfast meals in a cup are the ultimate in convenience—add boiling water and wait five minutes.

There are many varieties of rice. Long-grain rice, such as basmati, is higher in starch, so it cooks up separate and fluffy. Medium-grain rice, such as California, cooks up moist and tender. Short-grain rice is even softer and stickier than medium-grain rice.

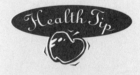

Whole grains cause faster weight loss than whole grain flour. Milling changes the physical properties, causing faster absorption of the carbohydrates, resulting in higher insulin levels, forcing fat into fat cells. Avoid breads, bagels, and pastas to lose faster.

Spicy Bulgur with Vegetables

Servings: 2 to 3
Preparation Time:
10 minutes
Cooking Time:
15 minutes
Resting Time:
5 minutes

1 cup bulgur
1¾ cups hot water
1½ cups spicy tomato juice
¼ cup lemon juice

3 zucchini
4 green onions, chopped
4 fresh basil leaves, chopped

Combine the bulgur and hot water in a saucepan and let rest for 5 minutes. Add the tomato juice and lemon juice, bring to a boil, and simmer over low heat for 15 minutes.

Meanwhile, cut the zucchini crosswise in thirds, then cut lengthwise in quarters. Place the zucchini in a microwave safe bowl and heat on high for 3 minutes, stirring once halfway through the cooking time.

Recipe Hint: To serve hot, place the zucchini on a plate alongside the spicy bulgur. Sprinkle the green onions and basil over the top. To serve cold, mix the zucchini, green onions, and basil into the spicy bulgur. Chill before serving.

Barleycorn Beans

Servings: 2
Preparation Time:
5 minutes
Cooking Time:
15 minutes

¾ cup water
½ cup quick-cooking barley
¼ cup chopped onion
¼ cup chopped bell pepper
1 cup frozen corn kernels, thawed

1 15-ounce can kidney beans, drained and rinsed
1 14.5-ounce can stewed tomatoes, Cajun, Mexican, or Italian-style

Place the water in a medium pot and bring to a boil. Add the barley, onion, and bell pepper. Mix well. When the mixture boils again, reduce heat, cover, and simmer over low heat for 12 minutes. Add the remaining ingredients and cook for another 3 minutes.

Gingered Green Grains

⅓ cup water
½ cup finely chopped onion
½ cup finely chopped green bell
  pepper
½ cup shredded carrot
2 teaspoons curry powder
1 teaspoon minced fresh garlic
1 teaspoon Sambal Oelek
½ teaspoon grated fresh gingerroot

2 cups cooked brown rice
1 cup cooked quinoa
1 15-ounce can garbanzo beans,
  drained and rinsed
1 tablespoon soy sauce
6 cups shredded kale or other
  leafy greens
2 tablespoons chopped
  cilantro

Servings: 4
Preparation Time:
10 minutes
(need cooked rice
and quinoa)
Cooking Time:
10 minutes

Place the water, onions, bell pepper, and carrots in a large non-stick frying pan. Cook, stirring frequently, for 4 minutes. Add the curry powder, garlic, Sambal Oelek, and ginger. Cook for 1 minute longer. Add the grains, beans, and soy sauce. Cook, stirring occasionally, for 2 minutes. Add the kale and cilantro and cook for an additional 3 minutes. Serve warm or at room temperature.

Recipe Hint: Use a food processor to shred the kale quickly. This is quite spicy because of the Sambal Oelek, a hot chili paste. If you don't like spicy foods, reduce the amount used by at least one half. This may also be made with barley in place of the rice.

Vegetable Paella

Servings: 4
Preparation Time:
15 minutes
Cooking Time:
25 minutes

⅓ cup water
1 onion, chopped
1½ teaspoons minced fresh garlic
4 cups vegetable broth
½ teaspoon white pepper
¼ teaspoon powdered saffron
1 cup arborio rice
2 cups cut green beans
2 zucchini, cut in half lengthwise, then sliced

1 red bell pepper, cut into strips
1 or 2 ears corn, cut into 1-inch pieces
1 tablespoon minced fresh basil
1 tablespoon minced fresh parsley
¼ teaspoon lemon zest
1 15-ounce can garbanzo beans, drained and rinsed
1 14-ounce can artichoke hearts, drained and rinsed

Place the water, onion, and garlic in a large saucepan. Cook, stirring frequently, for 3 minutes. Add the broth, pepper, and saffron. Bring to a boil and stir in the rice and green beans. Reduce heat, cover and cook over low heat for 8 minutes. Add the zucchini, bell pepper, corn, basil, parsley, and lemon zest. Mix well. Cover and cook for an additional 8 minutes. Add the garbanzo beans and artichoke hearts. Cook, stirring occasionally, for about 5 minutes. Serve hot.

Recipe Hint: This recipe can be varied by using different grains, but choose ones that cook in about 20 minutes. The pieces of corn can be pierced with a fork and the kernels bitten off, or pick them up with your fingers and eat them. If the artichoke hearts are very large, you may want to cut them in half before adding them to the pan.

HEALTHY SNACKS

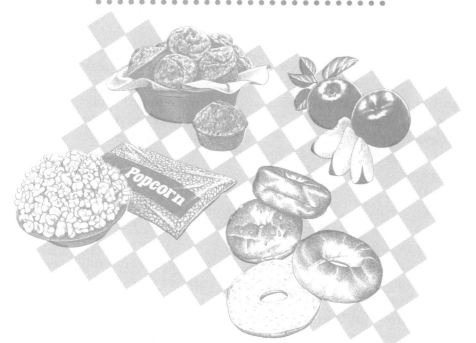

On the McDougall Program you are encouraged to eat to the full satisfaction of your appetite and to eat frequently, because studies show that nibblers, snackers, and grazers lose more weight and lower their cholesterol more than gorgers, who eat infrequently. In our home we have cups of instant soups, vegetables, bagels, baked fat-free tortilla chips and salsa, pretzels, fat-free potato chips, rice cakes, and whole grain crackers for snacking. Boiled red potatoes and canned, cooked garbanzo beans chase our hunger away.

Unless you have elevated triglycerides or are trying to lose weight, a bowl of fresh fruit on the kitchen counter is a great idea. Popcorn can be cooked in a microwave or an air popper, then seasoned with a light spray of soy sauce or sprinkled with brewer's yeast, chili powder, curry powder, onion powder, poultry seasoning, or paprika. Some of the healthiest snacks are leftovers from last night's dinner.

Don't get trapped by fat-free cakes and cookies. These are high sugar calorie bombs. Instead make your own healthy cookies, brownies, and bars using fat substitutes (Wonderslim and Just Like Shortenin'). Frozen juice popsicles or sorbet will replace that bowl of fat-laden ice cream you once snacked on before bedtime.

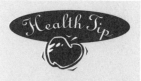

Health Tip

Insulin drives fat into fat cells, making you fat. Frequent small meals results in less insulin production than a few large meals. Alcohol, sugar, refined food, and diabetes medicine also raise insulin levels. Exercise and unrefined carbohydrates lower insulin levels.

Southwest Brown Rice

Servings: 4
Preparation Time:
10 minutes
Cooking Time:
10 minutes
Resting Time:
5 minutes

¼ cup water
1 onion, sliced and separated
  into rings
½ teaspoon minced fresh garlic
1 teaspoon ground cumin
1 teaspoon chili powder
1 14.5-ounce can stewed
  tomatoes

⅓ cup salsa or picante sauce
1 cup instant brown rice
1 15-ounce can kidney beans,
  drained and rinsed
1 small avocado, peeled and
  chopped (optional)

Place the water, onion, garlic, cumin, and chili powder in a large nonstick frying pan. Cook, stirring occasionally, for 2 to 3 minutes, until the onion softens.

Drain the stewed tomatoes and set aside; reserve the juice. Add enough water to the juice to make ¾ cup of liquid and add it to the onions along with the salsa or picante sauce. Bring to a boil, stir in the rice, cover, and cook over low heat for 5 minutes. Add the beans and tomatoes. Remove from heat and let rest for 5 minutes. Return to heat and cook until well heated, about 2 minutes. Serve with chopped avocado over the top, if desired.

Quick Curry Rice

1½ cups water
1 onion, chopped
1 garlic clove, minced
1 tablespoon curry
   powder

several twists of freshly ground
   black pepper
1½ cups instant brown rice
2 tomatoes, chopped
1 bunch green onions, chopped

Place ¼ cup of the water, the onion, and garlic in a saucepan and cook for about 5 minutes. Add the curry powder and pepper and the remaining 1¼ cups water. Bring to a boil, add the rice, reduce heat to low, cover, and simmer for 5 minutes. Remove from heat. Add the tomatoes and green onions. Mix, cover, and let rest for 5 more minutes. Toss gently before serving. Serve hot or cold.

Instant Mexican Rice

2½ cups water
2¼ cups instant brown rice
1 cup chopped green onions
1 green bell pepper,
   chopped

½ teaspoon minced fresh garlic
1 10-ounce can Ro-tel diced
   tomatoes and green chilies
½ cup salsa
¼ cup chopped cilantro

Bring 1¾ cups of the water to a boil in a saucepan. Stir in the rice. Return to a boil, cover, and cook over low heat for 5 minutes. Remove from heat, stir, cover, and let rest for 5 minutes.

Place the remaining ¾ cup water in another saucepan. Add the green onions, bell pepper, and garlic. Cook, stirring occasionally, for 10 minutes. Add the tomatoes and salsa. Stir in the hot rice and mix well. Cook until heated through. Stir in the cilantro and serve at once.

Recipe Hint: *To make this with leftover cooked brown rice, use 3 cups of cooked rice. Add to the vegetables at the same time you add the tomatoes and salsa.*

Servings: 4
Preparation Time:
10 minutes
Cooking Time:
15 minutes

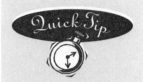

To remove the skin from a garlic clove, use one of the new garlic peelers sold in gourmet cooking stores or lay the clove flat on the counter and hit it with the side of a heavy knife—the skin will just slip off. Then use a garlic press to crush the garlic and a flat knife to remove minced garlic.

Servings: 4
Preparation Time:
15 minutes
Cooking Time:
15 minutes

Instant Fried Rice

Servings: 4
Preparation Time:
15 minutes
Cooking Time:
15 minutes

2 cups water
2¼ cups instant brown rice
3 tablespoons soy sauce
½ teaspoon minced fresh garlic
½ teaspoon minced fresh
   gingerroot

1 cup chopped green onions
1 cup broccoli florets
1 cup snow peas, cut in half
½ cup mung bean sprouts
½ cup shredded carrots

Bring 1¾ cups of the water to a boil. Stir in the rice. Return to a boil, cover, and simmer over low heat for 5 minutes. Remove from heat, stir, cover, and let rest for 5 minutes. Meanwhile, place the remaining ¼ cup water in another saucepan. Add 2 tablespoons of the soy sauce, the garlic, ginger, and vegetables. Cook, stirring frequently, for 10 minutes. Add the hot rice to the vegetables, mix well, add the remaining 1 tablespoon soy sauce, and mix again. Serve hot.

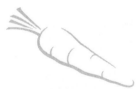

Recipe Hint: To make this with leftover brown rice, cook the vegetables as directed. After the vegetables have cooked, stir in 3 cups of cold brown rice and the remaining soy sauce. Cook until heated through.

THE MIXED FAMILY

+ = *harmony?*

| Don't prepare two meals | Add missing items | Substitute soy or seitan |

You're enthused about your new diet, but the rest of the family isn't. You need to set the example for everyone's sake. Do not make two separate meals. Instead, make your starch-based meal and add to it what your family thinks they're missing as side dishes. For example, make bean burritos for dinner. The main dish will be "refried" beans made without oil and whole wheat or corn tortilla shells. Put out bowls of lettuce, chopped tomatoes, onions, sprouts, and your favorite salsa sauces. To keep unconverted members happy, you might want to have on hand a bowl of grated cheese or seasoned ground beef. Make a meal of spaghetti and an oil-free marinara sauce, along with parmesan cheese and maybe some meatballs as side dishes to be added at the table. A plate of thinly sliced chicken added to your "fried" rice dish will keep harmony in the family. Experiencing healthier recipes will quickly bring about a change in family members' tastes.

Healthier meals can be made by using low-fat soy cheese, textured vegetable protein spiced with hamburger seasonings, and "meat" balls made from wheat gluten (seitan). You may want to use a little seitan and low-fat soy products every day to add a little richness to your dishes. In no time you will be able to conveniently forget to make the high-fat, high-cholesterol additions, and no one will protest.

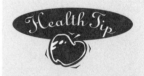

Health Tip

Our tastes for foods change with repeat exposure. Encourage everyone to at least try new healthy dishes; however, have at least one dish each person likes at each meal, even if it's only a simple dish, like rice or pasta. Enlist family members to help you plan the week's meals.

Spicy Arroz Verde

Servings: 4
Preparation Time:
10 minutes
Cooking Time:
25 minutes

2½ cups vegetable broth
1 cup chopped green onions
½ cup chopped green bell pepper
½ teaspoon minced fresh garlic
1 cup uncooked brown jasmine
   rice
2 tablespoons chopped canned
   green chilies

½ teaspoon ground cumin
½ teaspoon chili powder
freshly ground black pepper to
   taste
several dashes of Tabasco sauce
2 cups chopped fresh spinach
¼ cup chopped cilantro or
   parsley

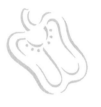

Place ½ cup of the vegetable broth into a saucepan. Add the green onions, bell pepper, and garlic. Cook, stirring occasionally, for 5 minutes. Add the remaining 2 cups vegetable broth, the rice, green chilies, cumin, chili powder, pepper, and Tabasco sauce. Bring to a boil, reduce heat, cover, and simmer for 15 minutes. Stir in the spinach, cover, and continue to cook for 5 more minutes, until the liquid is absorbed. Remove from heat and stir in the cilantro or parsley. Serve at once.

Rice Medley

½ cup vegetable broth
1 onion, chopped
1 green bell pepper, chopped
½ pound sliced fresh mushrooms
1 bunch green onions, chopped
½ teaspoon minced fresh garlic
1 14.5-ounce can stewed
   tomatoes

1 4-ounce can chopped green
   chilies
1 tablespoon soy sauce
1 teaspoon chili powder
dash or two of Tabasco sauce
4 cups cooked brown rice
¼ cup chopped cilantro

Servings: 6 to 8
Preparation Time:
15 minutes
(need cooked rice)
Cooking Time:
15 minutes

   Place the vegetable broth in a large pot. Add the onion, bell pepper, mushrooms, green onions, and garlic. Cook, stirring occasionally, for 5 minutes. Add the remaining ingredients, except the rice and cilantro. Cook, stirring occasionally, for 5 more minutes. Add the rice and cilantro. Cook for an additional 5 minutes. Serve at once.

Recipe Hint: Use one of the seasoned stewed tomatoes, such as Mexican-style, Cajun-style, or Italian-style, for even more flavor in this dish.

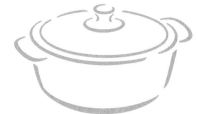

Bean and Rice Gumbo

Servings: 4 to 6
Preparation Time:
15 minutes
Cooking Time:
25 minutes

1 cup instant brown rice
1 onion, chopped
1 red bell pepper, chopped
1 yellow bell pepper, chopped
2 stalks celery, sliced
1 teaspoon minced fresh
   garlic
3½ cups vegetable broth

1 15-ounce can black beans,
   drained and rinsed
1 15-ounce can black-eyed peas,
   drained and rinsed
1 to 2 teaspoons Cajun
   seasoning mix
¼ teaspoon Tabasco sauce
1 cup frozen sliced okra

Prepare the rice according to package directions and set aside.
   Place the onion, bell peppers, celery, and garlic in a large pot with ½ cup of the broth. Cook, stirring occasionally, for 5 minutes. Add the remaining 3 cups broth, the beans, and seasonings. Bring to a boil, reduce heat, and simmer for 15 minutes. Add the okra and cook for an additional 5 minutes. Stir in the cooked rice. Serve at once.

Recipe Hint: *Cajun seasoning mix is a mixture of herbs and spices, often called blackening spice, and is usually found in gourmet cooking stores and sometimes supermarkets. You can make your own by mixing 3 tablespoons paprika, 2 teaspoons onion powder, 2 teaspoons black pepper, 2 teaspoons white pepper, 2 teaspoons cayenne, 1 teaspoon oregano, 1 teaspoon thyme, and ½ teaspoon celery seed. Use carefully! It can be very hot.*

Quinoa Surprise

1 cup vegetable broth
½ cup quinoa, rinsed
2 cups frozen peas, thawed
¾ cup chopped green onions
1 tomato, chopped
½ cup chopped cilantro

3 tablespoons lime juice
1 tablespoon soy sauce
several dashes of Tabasco sauce
freshly ground black pepper to
    taste

Servings: 4
Preparation Time:
10 minutes
Cooking Time:
10 minutes

Place the vegetable broth in a saucepan and bring to a boil. Add the quinoa. Cover, reduce heat, and simmer for 10 minutes. Remove from heat and set aside.

Combine the peas, green onions, tomato, and cilantro. Add the cooked quinoa and mix well. Add the remaining ingredients and toss well to mix. Serve warm or cold.

Recipe Hint: Quinoa must be rinsed before cooking to remove a bitter flavor. Quinoa (pronounced keen-wa) is a high-protein grain. Uncooked, it looks somewhat like toasted sesame seeds. It becomes translucent when cooked. It is available in natural food stores.

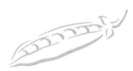

BREAST CANCER AND DIET

Rate: 100,000 Women

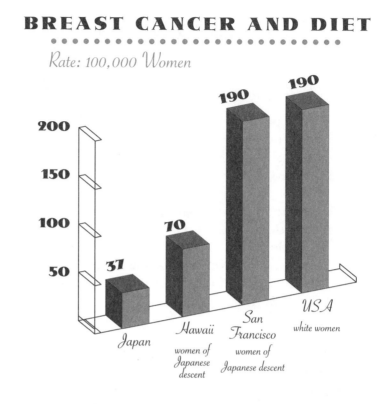

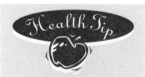

Health Tip

Even after a person has cancer, diet is very important. A healthy diet will cause them to live better and probably longer. After all, if you believe, like most experts, the high-fat American diet causes cancer, then it makes no sense to "throw gasoline on a fire."

Breast cancer is a woman's greatest fear. Worldwide, the incidence of breast cancer among women parallels their intake of rich foods. When people migrate, they take on the incidence of cancer of their new country, proving this is an environmental disease, not genetic. The strongest contact we have with our environment is our food.

Many qualities of this diet promote breast cancer. A rich diet is high in two recognized cancer promoters—fat and calories. Vegetable fats, such as safflower and corn oils, and animal protein suppress the immune system, and strongly promote cancer. Environmental chemicals concentrated in rich foods initiate and promote cancer. The rich Western diet also lacks substances that protect us from cancer. It is deficient in dietary fiber (found only in plants), vegetable substances that deactivate cancer-causing chemicals, plant-derived antioxidant vitamins (beta carotene, C, and E), that repair DNA damage, and compounds called phyto-estrogens that reduce the cancer-promoting effects of estrogen.

Savory Risotto

½ cup water
1 onion, chopped
1 cup sliced fresh mushrooms
1 green bell pepper, chopped
1 tomato, chopped
1 teaspoon minced fresh garlic
1 teaspoon crushed sage
¼ teaspoon thyme leaves

1½ cups arborio rice
5½ cups vegetable broth
1 15-ounce can black beans, drained and rinsed
freshly ground black pepper to taste
finely chopped cilantro to taste

Servings: 6
Preparation Time:
10 minutes
Cooking Time:
25 minutes

Place the water in a medium saucepan. Add the onion, mushrooms, bell pepper, tomato, garlic, sage, and thyme. Cook, stirring frequently, for 5 minutes. Stir in the rice and continue to cook for a minute or two.

Meanwhile, heat the vegetable broth to boiling in the microwave. Add the broth to the rice mixture. Cook, stirring occasionally, until the rice is cooked and the mixture is creamy, about 20 minutes. Stir in the beans and heat through. Add the pepper and sprinkle with the cilantro before serving.

Recipe Hint: *Arborio rice is an Italian rice that cooks to a smooth creaminess. You can find it in natural food stores and supermarkets. It is used in risottos because of its consistency.*

Vegetable Risotto

Servings: 6
Preparation Time:
15 minutes
Cooking Time:
15 minutes

3½ cups vegetable broth
1 cup arborio rice
½ cup water
1 onion, finely chopped
2 cups broccoli florets
1 cup finely chopped zucchini
1 cup frozen corn kernels, thawed

1 cup finely chopped red bell
   pepper
1 cup finely chopped green bell
   pepper
¼ cup finely chopped fresh basil
freshly ground black pepper to
   taste

Place the broth in a saucepan and bring to a boil. Stir in the rice, reduce heat, and cook over low heat, stirring frequently, until the broth is absorbed, about 15 minutes.

Meanwhile, place the water in a large nonstick frying pan. Add all the vegetables, except the basil. Cook, stirring occasionally, for 10 minutes. Remove from heat.

Combine the rice and vegetables. Stir in the basil. Season with the pepper.

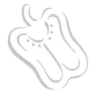

Slow Beans and Berries

Servings: 6 to 8
Preparation Time:
5 minutes
Cooking Time:
8 to 10 hours

5 cups water
1 cup great northern beans
¾ cup wheat berries
4 small red potatoes, cut in half
1 onion, sliced and separated
   into rings

2 teaspoons minced fresh
   garlic
4 teaspoons ground cumin
3 teaspoons turmeric
several twists of freshly ground
   black pepper

Combine all ingredients in a slow cooker. Cook for 8 to 10 hours on the high heat setting.

Recipe Hint: This is a delicious spicy stew that we have been making for more than 10 years. Wheat berries take a long time to get tender enough to chew, which makes them ideal for use in a slow cooker.

Vegetable Grain Casserole

1 cup vegetable broth
1 cup canned black beans, drained and rinsed
1 cup frozen corn kernels
1 cup thinly sliced carrots
1 cup sliced fresh mushrooms
½ cup barley

¼ cup bulgur
¼ cup chopped onion
2 tablespoons parsley flakes
½ teaspoon minced fresh garlic
½ cup shredded soy cheese (optional)

Servings: 6
Preparation Time: 15 minutes
Cooking Time: 60 minutes

Preheat the oven to 350 degrees.

Combine all ingredients, except the cheese, in a casserole dish. Cover and bake for 60 minutes, stirring once halfway through the cooking time. Sprinkle with cheese, if desired. Cover and let rest for 5 minutes.

Recipe Hint: *This may be prepared and baked ahead of time. Do not add the cheese until just before eating. It freezes well.*

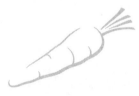

Barley Pilaf

⅓ cup water
1 onion, chopped
1 stalk celery, chopped
½ cup sliced fresh mushrooms
½ cup chopped red bell pepper
1 cup vegetable broth
½ cup quick-cooking barley

½ cup frozen corn kernels
½ cup frozen peas
¼ cup chopped fresh parsley
2 teaspoons chopped fresh basil or ½ teaspoon dried basil
several twists of freshly ground black pepper

Servings: 4
Preparation Time: 15 minutes
Cooking Time: 15 minutes

Place the water in a saucepan with the onion, celery, mushrooms, and bell pepper. Cook, stirring occasionally, for 3 minutes. Add the remaining ingredients. Bring to a boil, cover, reduce heat, and simmer for 12 minutes.

RAISING HEALTHY CHILDREN

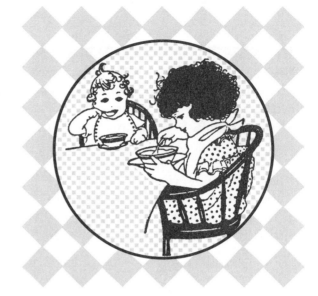

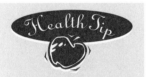

We believe bigger is better when it comes to our size. But consider that taller (and fatter) women have more breast cancer; and taller men and women have more colon cancer. The same over-nutrition that causes excess growth, also results in deadly diseases.

The most important legacy you can leave your children is good health. Habits begun early in life continue throughout life. Children need proper nutrients in order to grow. Breast-feeding is essential. Bottle-fed infants have at least twice the risk of crib death (SIDS) and five times the chance of serious illnesses leading to hospitalization during the first year of life, as well as a greater risk of developing obesity, allergies, diabetes, heart disease, multiple sclerosis, inflammatory bowel diseases (ulcerative colitis and Crohn's disease), acute appendicitis, tonsillitis, and cancer, especially lymphomas and acute leukemia. Bottle-fed babies have a lower IQ and poorer speech development. Mothers fully informed of the consequences of bottle-feeding would make every effort to provide their babies with the advantages of breast milk.

Children should be exclusively breast-fed until the age of six months. At about six months they develop their first teeth and the coordination to reach out for food on the table. That is the time to introduce solid foods. Cooked and mashed rice, potatoes, sweet potatoes, pasta, oatmeal, tofu, and fruits make excellent first foods. As the months go by increase the amount of solid food and decrease breast milk. Ideally, breast-feeding will continue until at least two years of age. Mothers who work may find a breast pump handy for later feeding.

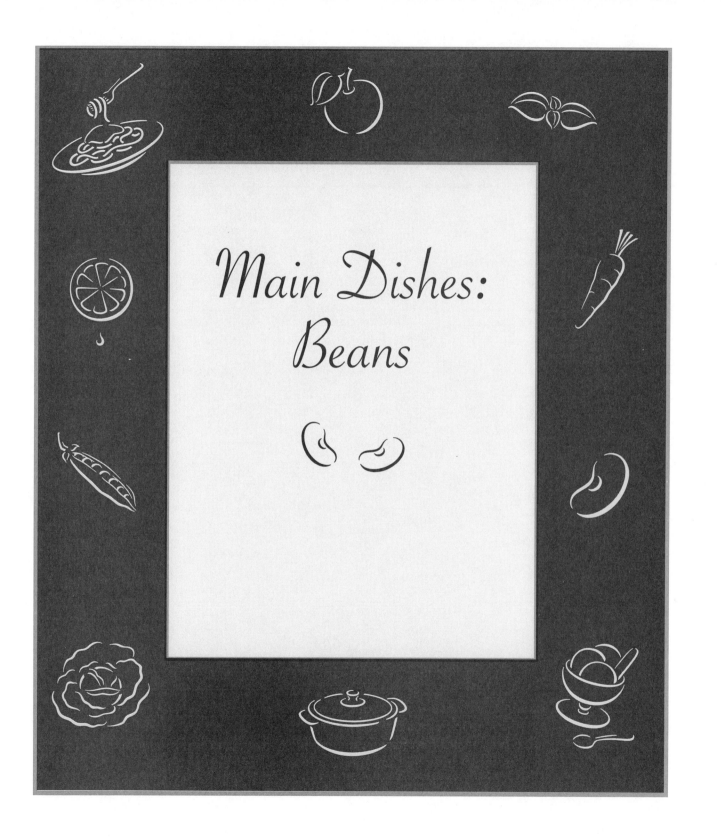

Main Dishes: Beans

Beans and Greens

2 15-ounce cans white beans, drained and rinsed

2 fresh ripe tomatoes, chopped

1 zucchini, cut in half lengthwise, then sliced

1 red bell pepper, thinly sliced

⅓ cup fat-free Italian dressing

2 tablespoons chopped fresh basil

freshly ground black pepper to taste

1 10-ounce bag mixed salad greens

Servings: 4
Preparation Time:
10 minutes

Combine all ingredients, except the salad greens, in a bowl. Toss well to mix. Place the greens in a large bowl. Add the vegetable mixture and toss to mix. Serve at once.

Recipe Hint: *Try other kinds of canned beans in this wonderful complete-meal salad. Serve on those hot summer days when you don't feel like cooking.*

Ten-Minute Chili

2 15-ounce cans kidney beans, drained and rinsed

2 cups fat-free spaghetti sauce

2 teaspoons chili powder

1 teaspoon ground cumin

dash of cayenne pepper (optional)

Servings: 4
Preparation Time:
5 minutes
Cooking Time:
10 minutes

Combine all ingredients in a saucepan and heat for 10 minutes, stirring occasionally. Ladle into bowls and serve.

Recipe Hint: *This simple recipe appeals to many children. Try serving it with baked tortilla chips to scoop up the chili.*

Disorderly Lentils

Servings: 6
Preparation Time:
15 minutes
Cooking Time:
30 minutes

2 cups red lentils
4 cups water
1 onion, chopped
1 green bell pepper, chopped
½ cup grated carrot
2 cups tomato sauce

2 tablespoons soy sauce
2 tablespoons parsley flakes
1 bay leaf
½ teaspoon chopped fresh
   garlic
½ teaspoon basil

Combine all ingredients in a medium pot. Bring to a boil, reduce heat, cover, and simmer for 30 minutes. Serve over toast, fat-free crumpets, fat-free English muffins, or whole wheat rolls.

Recipe Hint: This recipe could also be served over baked potatoes or grains. This recipe freezes well and reheats well.

Baked Beans and Dogs

Servings: 4
Preparation Time:
5 minutes
Cooking Time:
14 minutes

1 onion, chopped
⅓ cup water
2 16-ounce cans fat-free baked beans
1 15-ounce can red beans,
   drained and rinsed

2 tablespoons molasses
1 tablespoon prepared mustard
4 fat-free, meat-free hot dogs,
   sliced ½ inch thick

Place the onion and water in a saucepan. Cook, stirring occasionally, for 4 minutes. Add the remaining ingredients and cook for 10 minutes, until well heated.

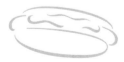

Recipe Hint: This is another favorite with kids. You can prepare it ahead and bake in the oven, if desired. Just cook the onion as directed, then combine the remaining ingredients in a casserole dish. Refrigerate until baking time. Bake at 350 degrees for 30 minutes.

KIDS' FAVORITES

All Vegetable Products

*C*hildren begin life liking simple meals—cold cereal, plain pasta, and mashed potatoes. Repeated exposures to salt- and sugar-laden foods soon pervert their tastes to breakfast sausages, lunch meats, hot dogs, cheese pizza, and ice cream. It may be a tough battle to get some kids back to healthy brown rice and vegetables. So don't try. Instead, find healthier substitutes for the foods they already like and emphasize their favorite starches, fruits, and vegetables.

Serve pancakes and waffles made of the right ingredients and sweeten with maple syrup but skip the butter. Hot and cold cereals with a sprinkle of sugar over the top will be a hit. Instead of cow's milk use rice, soy, almond, and cashew milks—they're white and taste sweet. For lunch make vegetable soups or bean and vegetable sandwiches. How about low-fat nonmeat hot dogs and hamburgers with whole wheat buns and all the trimmings—ketchup, mustard, pickle relish, and onions. Your kids will love them. For dinner make bean burritos, tostadas, spaghetti, and chili.

Offer your children a good dose of education on the importance of eating plant foods, along with these great eating experiences. Talk about their health, saving the environment, and avoiding animal suffering.

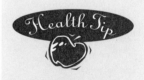

Vegetables are bursting with nutrients. Of the thirteen known vitamins, eleven are made by plants. One, vitamin D, is actually a hormone made by the action of sunlight on the skin. Vitamin B_{12} is made primarily by bacteria.

Bean Surprise

Servings: 6
Preparation Time:
15 minutes
Cooking Time:
15 minutes

⅓ cup water
1 onion, chopped
1 red bell pepper, chopped
1 green bell pepper, chopped
1 teaspoon minced fresh garlic
1 15-ounce can black beans, drained and rinsed
1 15-ounce can red beans, drained and rinsed

2 cups frozen corn kernels, thawed
1 15-ounce can stewed tomatoes (try Cajun, Mexican, or Italian)
1 tablespoon chili powder
freshly ground black pepper to taste

Place the water, onion, bell peppers, and garlic in a saucepan. Cook, stirring occasionally, for 5 minutes. Add the remaining ingredients and cook for another 10 minutes, stirring occasionally.

Recipe Hint: *These beans can be served any number of ways. Try them rolled up in burrito shells, on burger buns, or over grains, pasta, or baked potatoes.*

Cajun Black-Eyed Peas

⅓ cup water
1 onion, chopped
2 stalks celery, sliced
1 teaspoon minced fresh garlic
2 14-ounce cans Cajun-style
   stewed tomatoes
2 15-ounce cans black-eyed peas,
   drained and rinsed

2 tablespoons soy sauce
3 tablespoons ketchup
1 teaspoon paprika
½ teaspoon thyme
¼ teaspoon gumbo filé
⅛ teaspoon Tabasco sauce

Servings: 4
Preparation Time:
15 minutes
Cooking Time:
20 minutes

   Place the water, onion, celery, and garlic in a saucepan. Cook, stirring occasionally, for 5 minutes. Add the remaining ingredients. Cook, stirring occasionally, for 15 minutes.

Recipe Hint: *Serve over brown rice or another whole grain. Frozen black-eyed peas may be used in place of canned. Follow directions on the package for cooking. Gumbo filé is an ingredient often used in Southern cooking. It is made from sassafras leaves. It can be found in most supermarkets in the spice section.*

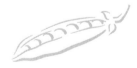

Spicy Chili and Chips

Servings: 6
Preparation Time:
10 minutes
Cooking Time:
20 minutes

Add dried bean flakes to soups and stews to thicken them and give them a bean-flavored broth. You can also use them to make instant "refried" beans for burritos.

⅓ cup water
1 onion, chopped
1 green bell pepper, chopped
1 teaspoon minced fresh garlic
1 15-ounce can kidney beans
1 14.5-ounce can chopped tomatoes
½ cup vegetable broth
¼ cup chopped canned green chilies
1 tablespoon parsley flakes
1 to 2 teaspoons chili powder
½ teaspoon ground cumin
freshly ground black pepper to taste
1 bag baked fat-free tortilla chips

Place the water in a pot with the onion, bell pepper, and garlic. Cook, stirring occasionally, for 5 minutes. Add the remaining ingredients, except the chips. Cook, stirring occasionally, for 15 minutes. Serve in a bowl with chips on the side to scoop up the chili.

Quick Wisconsin Chili

Servings: 4 to 6
Preparation Time:
7 minutes
Cooking Time:
25 minutes

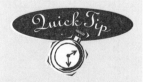

Frozen already-cut onions are found in your supermarket (Ore-Ida brand, for example). Add them frozen to your recipes and cook.

5 cups water
1 cup uncooked elbow macaroni
1 15-ounce can fat-free organic tomato soup
1 15-ounce can kidney beans, drained and rinsed
1 14.5-ounce can chopped tomatoes
½ cup chopped onions
½ cup chopped green bell pepper
2 teaspoons chili powder
freshly ground black pepper to taste

Place the water in a large pot and bring to a boil. Add the macaroni and cook for 5 minutes. Add the remaining ingredients and cook for 20 minutes, stirring occasionally. Add more water if necessary to keep a thick-soup consistency.

Tri-Bean Barbecue

1 onion, chopped
1 teaspoon minced fresh garlic
⅓ cup water
⅓ cup ketchup
1 tablespoon cider vinegar
1 tablespoon Sucanat
2 teaspoons Dijon-style mustard

1 15-ounce can fat-free
   vegetarian beans in tomato
   sauce
1 15-ounce can kidney beans,
   drained and rinsed
1 15-ounce can black beans,
   drained and rinsed

Servings: 6
Preparation Time:
10 minutes
Cooking Time:
45 minutes

Preheat oven to 375 degrees.

Place the onion and garlic in a small saucepan with the water. Cook, stirring occasionally until softened, about 5 minutes.

Combine the ketchup, vinegar, Sucanat, and mustard in a small bowl.

Combine the beans in another bowl. Mix all ingredients together and pour into an uncovered baking dish. Bake for 40 minutes, stirring occasionally.

__Recipe Hint:__ Sucanat is granulated cane juice. It is made from sugarcane juice. Nothing is added, only water is removed, retaining all the vitamins, minerals, and trace elements. Sold in natural food stores, it may be used to replace white or brown sugar in recipes in equal amounts.

LEGUMES—FAST & EASY

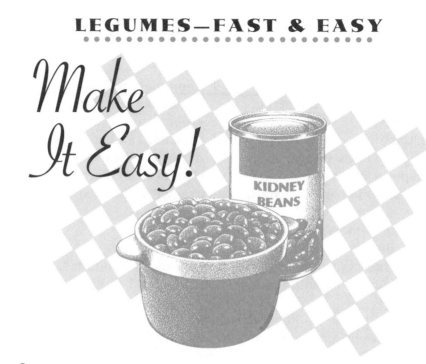

Make It Easy!

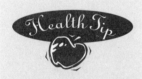

Legumes include beans, peas, and lentils. They are easy to cook on a stovetop or in a slow cooker or pressure cooker. Before cooking, sort beans by hand to remove stones. Most beans cook in one and a half to three hours; split peas and lentils take about an hour. The longer you cook them, the softer they get, and the less trouble they cause with bowel gas. Cooking times can be reduced by soaking overnight. Slow cookers take six to eight hours on high and ten to twelve hours on low to cook legumes. The best way to make your own home-cooked legumes fast and easy is to make large amounts and freeze them in meal-size plastic containers.

Precooked legumes can be bought in bottles and cans. Peas and black-eyed peas are available frozen in bags. Packaged products are more expensive but save time and energy for cooking.

Bowel gas is produced when carbohydrates not absorbed by your intestine are digested by gas-forming bacteria in your large intestine. To avoid bothersome gas, don't eat legumes or cook them thoroughly to help break down the indigestible carbohydrates. You can also cover them with water for twelve hours, then drain and spread on a moist towel, and let sprout for twelve hours before cooking. Or take a packaged digestive enzyme product called Beano or activated charcoal after meals.

Black-eyed Susans

1 small onion, chopped
1 green bell pepper, chopped
½ teaspoon minced fresh garlic
⅓ cup water
2 15-ounce cans black beans,
  drained and rinsed

1½ cups frozen corn kernels,
  thawed
¾ teaspoon ground cumin
¾ teaspoon ground coriander
1 tablespoon chopped fresh
  cilantro

Servings: 4
Preparation Time:
10 minutes
Cooking Time:
10 minutes

Place the onion, bell pepper, and garlic in a medium saucepan with the water. Cook, stirring frequently, over medium heat for 5 minutes. Add the remaining ingredients and cook for 5 more minutes. May be served warm or cold.

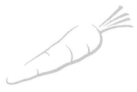

Beans Florentine

1 onion, chopped
1 stalk celery, chopped
1 carrot, chopped
1 teaspoon minced fresh garlic
½ cup water
3 15-ounce cans white beans
1 cup vegetable broth

1 tablespoon soy sauce
1 teaspoon dried basil
1 teaspoon dried oregano
freshly ground black pepper to
  taste
2 cups chopped fresh spinach

Servings: 6
Preparation Time:
10 minutes
Cooking Time:
28 minutes

Place the onion, celery, carrot, and garlic in a large pot with the water. Cook, stirring occasionally, for 5 minutes. Add the beans, broth, soy sauce, basil, oregano, and pepper. Cook over low heat for 20 minutes. Add the spinach and cook for 3 minutes longer. Serve over grains, potatoes, toast, or English muffins.

Crushing herbs releases flavor. Crush dried herbs in the palm of your hand with the fingers of your other hand. Use a mortar and pestle for hard herbs like rosemary and fennel seeds.

Black-eyed Pea Scramble

Servings: 6
Preparation Time:
5 minutes
Cooking Time:
10 minutes

1 15-ounce can black-eyed peas, drained and rinsed
1½ cups frozen chopped hash brown potatoes
1 onion, chopped
3 tablespoons ketchup or barbecue sauce

1 teaspoon Worcestershire sauce
½ teaspoon oregano
½ teaspoon thyme
freshly ground black pepper to taste

Place the peas, potatoes, and onion in a saucepan with water to cover. Cover and cook over medium heat until the potatoes are tender, about 10 minutes. Drain. Add the remaining ingredients and heat through. Serve stuffed into pita bread, rolled up in a tortilla, or spooned over toasted whole wheat bread or rolls.

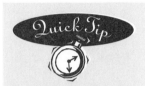

Quick Tip

One of our favorite uses of oil-free barbecue sauce is with packaged oil-free frozen hash brown potatoes for breakfast (and sometimes dinner). A tiny bit adds lots of flavor to recipes. Try a barbecue sauce instead of ketchup on fat-free vegetable burgers or hot dogs.

Fast Refried Beans

Servings:
makes 4 cups
Preparation Time:
5 minutes
Cooking Time:
10 minutes

2 16-ounce cans fat-free refried beans
½ cup mild salsa

½ teaspoon onion powder
¼ teaspoon garlic powder

Combine all ingredients in a saucepan and cook over low heat about 10 minutes to blend the flavors.

Recipe Hint: Precooked and even fat-free refried beans can be found in every supermarket. There are black, white, red, kidney, and pinto beans. Use them for "almost instant burritos and tortillas" made by spreading whole or mashed beans on a corn or whole wheat tortilla and adding tomatoes, onions, sprouts, and your favorite salsa. Use cooked whole beans for the foundation of cold salads or add them to soups and stews.

Barbecued Beans and Rice

1¼ cups water
1 small onion, chopped
1 red bell pepper, chopped
1 15.5-ounce can black beans,
    drained and rinsed
1 15.5-ounce can garbanzo beans,
    drained and rinsed
1 15.5-ounce can kidney beans,
    drained and rinsed

1 15.5-ounce can red beans,
    drained and rinsed
1 14.5-ounce can stewed
    tomatoes
½ cup oil-free barbecue sauce
2 cups cooked brown rice

Servings: 6 to 8
Preparation Time:
10 minutes
(need cooked rice)
Cooking Time:
15 minutes

Place ¼ cup of the water, the onion, and bell pepper in a large saucepan. Cook, stirring occasionally, for 5 minutes. Add the remaining ingredients, except the rice. Cook for 10 minutes. Stir in the rice and heat through.

Recipe Hint: *This freezes well. Use Cajun, Mexican, or Italian stewed tomatoes for a change in flavor.*

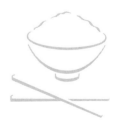

PROBLEMS WITH VEGETABLE OIL

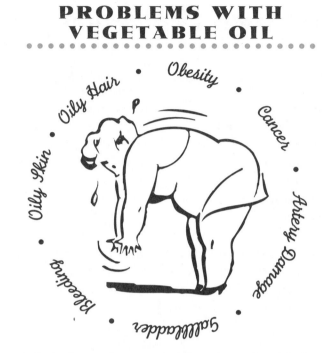

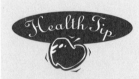

Health Tip

There has never been a case of fat deficiency in human beings caused by eating a low-fat diet. Vegetable foods contain generous amounts of essential fats; for example, rice is 5 percent, corn is 8 percent, and oatmeal is 16 percent fat.

Many people believe that vegetable oil is a health food because it lowers cholesterol and reduces the risk of dying of heart disease. However, choosing between animal fat and vegetable oil is like choosing between being shot or being hanged.

Like animal fats, vegetable fats are easily stored by your body. Vegetable oils are stronger promoters of cancer than lard (particularly corn and safflower oils) and have been found to damage the arteries as much as animal fat (even olive oil). The incidence of heart disease is less common because the blood is "thinned" by the vegetable fats, reducing the likelihood of blood clot formation in heart arteries, which can lead to a heart attack. However, your "thinned" blood makes you more likely to bleed to death if you are involved in an accident. When men in the Veterans Administration Hospital Study were switched from animal to vegetable fats, their cholesterol levels fell, and they had less chance of dying from heart disease. But their overall death rate was the same with more cancer and gallbladder disease.

Vegetable fats, like animal fats, are deposited on the skin. Your veterinarian recommends adding eggs, lard, or vegetable oil to your dog's food to make his coat shiny. A shiny coat on a dog is attractive, but greasy hair and faces are unattractive on people.

Baked Beans

1 onion, chopped
1 green bell pepper, chopped
1 red bell pepper, chopped
3 cans red beans

½ cup brown sugar, firmly
    packed
⅓ cup prepared mustard
¼ cup molasses

Combine the vegetables and beans in a bowl. Combine the remaining ingredients in a separate bowl. Pour over the beans and vegetables and mix well. Pour into a casserole dish, cover, and bake for 1 hour.

Servings: 6
Preparation Time:
15 minutes
Cooking Time:
1 hour

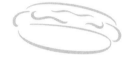

Beans and Franks

1 cup water
1 zucchini, diced
1 cup frozen diced hash brown
    potatoes

¾ cup frozen corn kernels
2 15-ounce cans black beans
3 fat-free, meat-free hot dogs
¼ cup oil-free barbecue sauce

Place the water in a medium pot. Add the zucchini, potatoes, and corn. Cook over medium heat for 5 minutes. Add the remaining ingredients. Cook, uncovered, over medium heat for 20 minutes, stirring occasionally. Serve as a stew or use over baked potatoes, toast, or whole grains.

Servings: 6
Preparation Time:
10 minutes
Cooking Time:
25 minutes

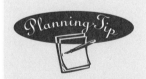

Plan meals as one main dish, with at most a simple side dish: for example, a bean soup and bread, or pasta with marinara sauce and a green salad. Resist the temptation to have four-course meals—few people will appreciate your efforts.

Recipe Hint: *There are many varieties of fat-free, meat-free hot dogs available in natural food stores. See the canned and packaged products list on page 286 for some suggestions.*

Italian Bean Medley

Servings: 6
Preparation Time:
10 minutes
Cooking Time:
28 minutes

1 onion, chopped
⅓ cup water
½ teaspoon minced fresh garlic
2 15-ounce cans white beans, drained and rinsed

2 15-ounce cans Italian-style stewed tomatoes
1 zucchini, chopped
1 green bell pepper, chopped
1 cup frozen lima beans

Place the onion, water, and garlic in a medium pot. Cook, stirring occasionally, for 3 minutes. Add the remaining ingredients. Cover and cook over medium heat for 25 minutes.

Irish Bean Stew

Servings: 6
Preparation Time:
15 minutes
Cooking Time:
24 minutes

1 onion, chopped
⅓ cup water
¾ teaspoon caraway seeds
2 cups frozen chopped hash brown potatoes
2 cups frozen mixed vegetables

1¾ cups vegetable broth
4 cups coarsely chopped cabbage
2 15-ounce cans white beans
freshly ground black pepper to taste

Place the onion and water in a large pot. Cook, stirring frequently, for 3 minutes. Add the caraway seeds and cook and stir for another minute. Add the potatoes, mixed vegetables, and vegetable broth. Mix well, cover, and cook for 5 minutes. Stir in the cabbage and cook for another 5 minutes. Add the beans and cook for 10 minutes longer, stirring occasionally. Season with the pepper. Serve in a bowl.

Recipe Hint: You don't have to thaw the frozen vegetables before using them in this recipe. As the potatoes cook, they thicken the stew. This is a delicious dish for a cool winter evening. Whenever we make it there are never any leftovers. We like to eat this with slices of bread to dunk into the broth.

Southwest Four-Bean Chili

¼ cup water
1 onion, chopped
3 stalks celery, chopped
1 15-ounce can kidney beans,
    drained and rinsed
1 15-ounce can black beans,
    drained and rinsed
1 15-ounce can white beans,
    drained and rinsed

2 14.5-ounce cans Mexican-style
    stewed tomatoes
1 cup each frozen corn kernels
    and frozen lima beans
1 tablespoon lime juice
2 teaspoons chili powder
2 teaspoons ground cumin
¼ cup chopped cilantro
    (optional)

Servings: 8
Preparation Time:
10 minutes
Cooking Time:
25 minutes

Place the water in a large pot with the onion and celery. Cook, stirring occasionally, for 5 minutes. Add the remaining ingredients, except the cilantro. Cover and cook over medium heat for 20 minutes. Stir in the cilantro, if desired, and serve at once.

Recipe Hint: *This is delicious over baked potatoes, rolled up in a tortilla, stuffed into pita bread, or served in a bowl with a loaf of bread on the side to dunk in the sauce.*

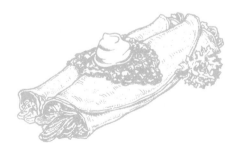

SAUTEING WITHOUT OIL

Oil-free Salad Dressing
Vinegar/Fruit Juice
Soy Sauce
Tomato/Vegetable Juice
Barbecue Sauce
Salsa
Water with herbs/spices

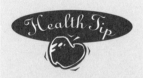

Health Tip

Natural oils found in plant foods are protected from rancidity by their surrounding environment of vitamins, minerals, and phytochemicals. Free oils spoil quickly. Rancidity produces "free radicals" that damage your arteries causing atherosclerosis and also damage your DNA causing cancer.

Mary once believed that vegetables had to be cooked in oil to turn brown. Not so. Water is an excellent medium for sautéing vegetables. For example, place chopped onions in a nonstick frying pan and cover with water. Cook, stirring frequently, until all the water has evaporated. Loosen the onions from the bottom of the pan. Add more water and repeat the process until the onions are as brown as you like. The slow heating not only brings out the sweet taste of the onion by slowing the breakdown of the carbohydrates into simple sugars but also removes gaseous substances that commonly cause indigestion when people eat raw onions. Any other vegetable can be browned using the same technique.

Other flavorful liquids can also be used to sauté and brown vegetables. Try vegetable broth, oil-free salad dressings, soy sauce, barbecue sauce mixed with a little water, vinegar, fruit juice, tomato juice, salsa, or water with herbs. In most of the recipes in this book the vegetables are cooked in a small amount of water or vegetable broth.

Quick Spicy Lentil Chili

2 cups red lentils
2 quarts vegetable broth
2 cups diced onion
1 16-ounce can chopped
  tomatoes
¼ cup tomato paste
2 tablespoons chopped fresh
  garlic
2 tablespoons balsamic vinegar
2 tablespoons fresh lime juice

1 tablespoon ground cumin
1 tablespoon chili powder
1 teaspoon paprika
½ teaspoon thyme
several twists of freshly ground
  black pepper
pinch of crushed red pepper
dash of cayenne pepper
¼ cup chopped fresh cilantro

Servings: 8
Preparation Time:
15 minutes
Cooking Time:
30 to 35 minutes

Combine all of the ingredients, except the cilantro, in a large soup pot. Bring to a boil over high heat. Reduce the heat, cover, and simmer over medium-low heat for 30 to 35 minutes, until the lentils are tender, stirring occasionally, adding more water or broth if needed for proper chili consistency. Remove from heat, stir in the cilantro, and serve.

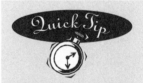

Thicken soups (and some-times stews) with instant mashed potatoes. Buy a brand made from dehy-drated potatoes—no milk, no eggs.

Beans and Things

Servings: 6
Preparation Time:
15 minutes
Cooking Time:
1 hour

2 15-ounce can white beans,
    drained and rinsed
2 cups chopped broccoli
1 cup chopped cauliflower
1 onion, chopped
1 rib celery, chopped
½ cup chopped carrots

1 large tomato, chopped
2 tablespoons soy sauce
1½ tablespoons molasses
2 teaspoons chili powder
2 teaspoons basil
⅛ teaspoon cayenne pepper

Preheat the oven to 350 degrees.

Combine the beans and vegetables in a large bowl. Combine the remaining ingredients in a small bowl and pour over the vegetable mixture; mix well. Pour into a casserole dish, cover, and bake for 1 hour. Serve plain or rolled up in corn or flour tortillas.

> **Recipe Hint:**   *This seems like a lot of ingredients, but the dish is really very easy to put together, and it tastes delicious. To save time, buy cleaned chopped broccoli and cauliflower and small cleaned carrots.*

Vegetable Bean Casserole

½ cup water
1 small onion, chopped
1 small red bell pepper, chopped
1 zucchini, chopped
1 yellow summer squash, chopped
½ teaspoon minced fresh garlic

1 15-ounce can fat-free chili beans or baked beans
¾ cup frozen corn kernels
1 teaspoon parsley flakes
¼ teaspoon thyme
¼ teaspoon oregano
¼ cup grated soy cheese

Servings: 6
Preparation Time:
10 minutes
Cooking Time:
22 minutes

Preheat the oven to 350 degrees.

Place the water in a large saucepan. Add the onion, red pepper, zucchini, squash, and garlic. Cook, stirring frequently, for 7 minutes. Add the beans, corn, and seasonings. Heat through, about 5 minutes. Pour into a casserole dish. Top with the grated cheese. Cover and bake for 10 minutes.

Use a food processor to shred onions, carrots, celery, peppers, mushrooms, zucchini, kale, parsley, and cilantro into bite-size pieces in seconds.

Black Bean Sloppy Joes

Servings: 6
Preparation Time:
10 minutes
Cooking Time:
10 minutes

1 onion, chopped
1 green bell pepper, diced
⅓ cup water
1 15-ounce can black beans,
    drained and rinsed
1 8-ounce can tomato sauce

¼ cup quick-cooking oatmeal
1 tablespoon soy sauce
½ tablespoon prepared mustard
1 teaspoon honey
1 teaspoon chili powder
6 whole wheat buns

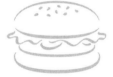

Place the onion and bell pepper in a saucepan with the water. Cook, stirring frequently, until the vegetables soften, about 5 minutes.

Meanwhile, mash the beans with a bean or potato masher (do not use a food processor). Add the beans and remaining ingredients, except the buns. Cook over low heat until heated through, about 5 minutes.

Serve on the buns with your choice of accompaniments, such as onions, tomatoes, lettuce, pickles, mustard, and ketchup.

Recipe Hint: Try this over toast, potatoes, or grains. Canned pinto beans also work well in this recipe.

DON'T GET SUCKERED

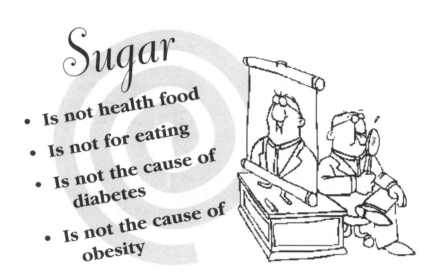

Sugar

- **Is not health food**
- **Is not for eating**
- **Is not the cause of diabetes**
- **Is not the cause of obesity**

*Y*ou avoided sugar and still got fatter. You used artificial sweeteners on your cereals and in your coffee and you gained. You order a diet coke with your cheeseburger and your weight goes up. Why? Sugar has very little to do with fat gain. Carbohydrates provide our body with energy. Excess carbohydrate (about two pounds) is stored invisibly in the muscles and liver as glycogen, or eliminated from the body as heat. It is too wasteful for the body to turn excess carbohydrate into fat. However, fat is easily stored.

Likewise, sugar has been the scapegoat for diabetes. More than 70 years ago doctors knew that fat paralyzed insulin activity and caused diabetes. Research has also shown how carbohydrates, even pure white sugar, make insulin work better (by increasing insulin sensitivity). Doctors have been successfully treating adult-onset diabetes for more than fifty years with a high-carbohydrate, low-fat diet. Research has shown that nearly two thirds of patients with adult-type diabetes can stop their insulin, and almost always stop diabetes pills, by changing their diet and by exercising.

Don't get suckered into believing sugar causes diabetes (or obesity). However, sugar is not health food. Sugar rots teeth, raises triglycerides in sensitive people, and causes serious nutritional imbalances when large amounts are consumed.

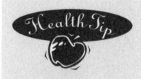

Health Tip

People with diabetes have a serious metabolic handicap—they can't defend themselves from disease as well—for example, a small cut can lead to gangrene. When it comes to food, they need to eat the best foods to keep their heart, kidneys, and eyes working into old age.

Louisiana Red Beans

Servings: 6
Preparation Time:
15 minutes
Cooking Time:
20 minutes

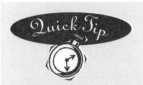

Nonstick-coated rice cookers cook your rice perfectly every time and keep it hot. Brown rice takes more water to cook. Try putting the water in first and then a cup of rice to get the correct amount of water.

½ cup water
1 onion, chopped
1 green bell pepper, chopped
2 stalks celery, chopped
1 teaspoon minced fresh garlic
3 15-ounce cans red beans, undrained
1 8-ounce can tomato sauce

2 bay leaves
1 teaspoon Tabasco sauce
1 teaspoon chili powder
1 teaspoon paprika
½ teaspoon thyme
¼ teaspoon ground cumin
1 to 2 pinches cayenne pepper

Place the water in a large sauce pot. Add the onion, bell pepper, celery, and garlic. Cook, stirring frequently, for 10 minutes. Add the remaining ingredients and cook for another 10 minutes. Serve over brown rice.

Slow-Cooked Lentil Stew

Servings: 4 to 6
Preparation Time:
10 minutes
Cooking Time:
4 hours

2 cups lentils
5 cups V8 juice
1 onion, chopped
1 carrot, thinly sliced
2 stalks celery with tops, sliced

1 16-ounce can stewed tomatoes
½ teaspoon minced fresh garlic
½ teaspoon oregano
¼ teaspoon black pepper

Place all ingredients in a slow cooker and cook on high for 4 hours, or on low for 8 hours.

Peppered Black Beans and Sausage

*Servings: 6
Preparation Time:
15 minutes
Cooking Time:
20 minutes*

1 onion, chopped
1 green bell pepper, chopped
⅓ cup water
1 teaspoon minced fresh garlic
3 15-ounce cans black beans,
    drained and rinsed
1 15-ounce can tomato sauce
1½ teaspoons oregano

1½ teaspoons basil
1 teaspoon white pepper
¼ teaspoon cayenne pepper
several twists of freshly ground
    black pepper
6 nonfat, meat-free hot dogs or
    sausages

Place the onion, bell pepper, water, and garlic in a large saucepan. Cook, stirring frequently, for 5 minutes. Add the remaining ingredients and cook over low heat for 15 minutes, stirring occasionally.

Recipe Hint: *This may also be made in a slow cooker. Add all ingredients at once. Cook on low for 8 hours or on high for 4 hours.*

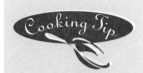

Put your vegetable stew or soup ingredients in a slow cooker before you leave for work. Before going to bed at night, add water to whole grains and dried fruits, and a hot breakfast awaits you in the morning.

Williams Crock Pot Chili

Servings: 8 to 10
Preparation Time:
15 minutes
Cooking Time:
4 hours

1 large onion, chopped
1½ teaspoons minced fresh
  garlic
⅓ cup water
2 tablespoons vegetable broth
  powder
2 tablespoons honey
1 tablespoon red wine vinegar
1 tablespoon paprika
½ tablespoon chili powder

½ teaspoon ground cumin
½ teaspoon cinnamon
¼ teaspoon nutmeg
2 15-ounce cans white beans
2 15-ounce cans black beans
1 15-ounce can red or pinto
  beans
1 15-ounce can black-eyed peas
1 15-ounce can chopped
  tomatoes

Place the onion, garlic, and water in a small saucepan. Cook, stirring occasionally, for 3 minutes. Add all the seasonings, mix well, and heat for 1 minute. Combine the beans and tomatoes in a Crock Pot. Add the onion-seasoning mixture, mix well, cover, and cook on high for 4 hours.

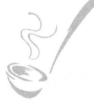

Recipe Hint: *This may also be cooked on low for 8 to 10 hours, so you could prepare it in the morning before leaving for the day and come home to a delicious, ready-to-eat meal.*

Slow-Cooked Bean Toppings

One

1 cup dried split peas
½ cup dried lima beans
½ cup dried white beans or
  garbanzos
1 onion, chopped

½ teaspoon minced fresh garlic
2 teaspoons dried basil
1 bay leaf
4 cups water

Two

1 cup dried kidney beans
½ cup dried pinto beans
½ cup dried white beans
1 onion, chopped
½ teaspoon minced fresh garlic

½ teaspoon chili powder
½ teaspoon ground cumin
¼ teaspoon ground oregano
4 cups water

Servings: 8
Preparation Time:
5 minutes
Cooking Time:
8 to 10 hours

Add all ingredients from either One or Two to your slow cooker. Stir. Cover and cook for 8 to 10 hours on high.

Recipe Hint: *These mixtures freeze well and are good for a fast meal. Try these delicious toppings poured over toast, rice, or potatoes. We have cooked them overnight and we eat them for breakfast over toast.*

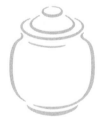

THE HAZARDS OF NONFAT DAIRY PRODUCTS

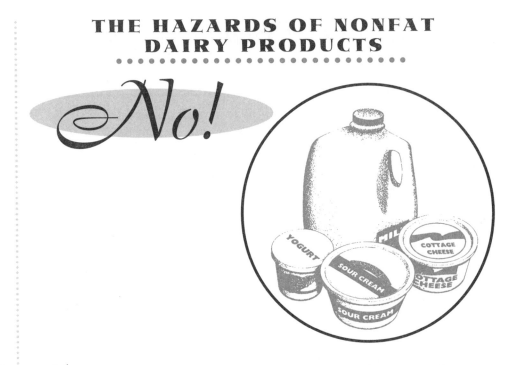

No!

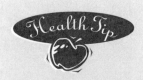

Dairy products should be thought of as "liquid meat." They have similar amounts of cholesterol and fat, and like meats, have no dietary fiber. One way they differ is milk has virtually no iron, and meat essentially no calcium.

High-fat dairy products cause obesity, heart disease, and cancer, so most of us have switched to low-fat and nonfat products and now think we're eating health food. Wrong! When you take the fat out of dairy products, you increase the relative concentrations of two other troublesome ingredients: milk protein and milk sugar.

Cow's milk protein is the leading cause of food allergies that include snotty nose, ear infections, asthma, bed-wetting, and eczema. It can also cause more serious, life-threatening immune problems, known as autoimmune diseases, such as childhood diabetes and glomerulonephritis (kidney disease). The number-one cause of anemia in children is cow's milk. Milk has almost no iron, and the calcium and phosphorus in milk form complexes with iron from other food sources (like green beans or beef) and prevent its absorption, and cow's milk protein causes the child's intestine to bleed. Cow's milk can be infected with bacteria, such as salmonella, Listeria, E coli, and tuberculosis. Bovine AIDS and bovine leukemia viruses infect more than 60 percent of the dairy herds in the United States. The high animal protein content of nonfat dairy products causes calcium loss, which contributes to kidney stones and osteoporosis. Lactose, the milk sugar in nonfat milk, is not digested by most adults and causes stomach cramps, gas, and diarrhea.

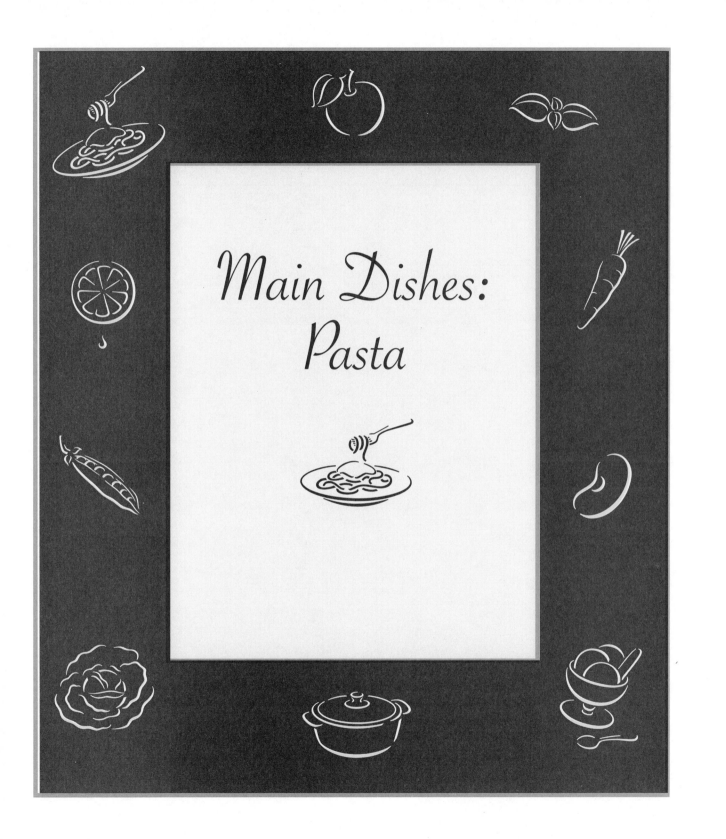

Main Dishes: Pasta

Curried Couscous

1 onion, chopped
¼ cup water
½ cup slivered almonds
½ cup raisins

1½ teaspoons curry powder
3¼ cups vegetable broth
2 cups couscous

Place the onion and water in a medium pot. Cook, stirring frequently, for 3 minutes. Add the almonds and raisins. Cook for another minute. Add the curry powder and vegetable broth. Bring to a boil. Stir in the couscous, cover, and remove from heat. Let rest for 5 minutes, until the liquid has been absorbed. Fluff with a fork before serving.

Moroccan Couscous

½ cup water
1 onion, chopped
1 carrot, thinly sliced
1 green bell pepper, chopped
1 tomato, chopped
½ teaspoon ground cumin
¼ teaspoon cinnamon
¼ teaspoon turmeric
1 15-ounce can garbanzo beans, drained and rinsed

4 green onions, chopped
2 tablespoons chopped canned green chilies
3 cups vegetable broth
2 cups couscous
¼ cup chopped fresh parsley
freshly ground black pepper to taste

Place the water in a large saucepan. Add the onion, carrot, bell pepper, and tomato. Cook, stirring occasionally, for 5 minutes. Add the spices and mix well. Add the remaining ingredients, except for the parsley and pepper. Bring to a boil, cover, remove from heat, and let rest for 5 minutes. Stir in the parsley and pepper. Serve at once.

Servings: 6 to 8
Preparation Time:
5 minutes
Cooking Time:
10 minutes

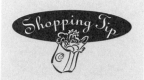

Shopping Tip

Buy large bags of beans, peas, lentils, grains, and potatoes. Store beans and grains in airtight bottles. Store all vegetables and grains in cool dry places.

Servings: 6
Preparation Time:
10 minutes
Cooking Time:
15 minutes

Black and Yellow Couscous

Servings: 4
Preparation Time:
10 minutes
Cooking Time:
10 minutes

1½ cups water
1 cup couscous
¼ cup orange juice
¼ cup lemon juice
1 tablespoon soy sauce
¼ teaspoon ground cumin
several twists of freshly ground
    black pepper

dash or two of Tabasco sauce
1 15-ounce can black beans,
    drained and rinsed
1½ cups frozen corn kernels,
    thawed
½ cup chopped fresh parsley or
    cilantro
¼ cup chopped green onions

Bring the water to a boil in a medium saucepan. Stir in the couscous. Cover and remove from heat. Let rest for 5 minutes. Fluff with a fork.

Meanwhile, combine the orange juice, lemon juice, soy sauce, cumin, pepper, and Tabasco. Set aside.

Place the couscous, beans, corn, parsley or cilantro, and green onions in a bowl. Toss to mix. Pour the sauce over and toss again. Serve warm or cold.

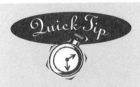

Quick Tip

To thaw frozen vegetables quickly, place in a colander and hold under cold running water. Shake off the excess water and use.

Spicy Tomato Couscous

Servings: 4 to 6
Preparation Time:
10 minutes
Cooking Time:
20 minutes

1¾ cups vegetable broth
1 cup couscous
1 onion, chopped
1 bunch green onions, chopped
1 teaspoon minced fresh garlic
1 28-ounce can chopped
    tomatoes

2 teaspoons basil
1 teaspoon thyme
¼ teaspoon crushed red
    pepper
¼ teaspoon Tabasco sauce
freshly ground black pepper to
    taste

Place 1½ cups of the vegetable broth into a saucepan. Bring to a boil and add the couscous. Mix well, cover, and remove from heat. Set aside.

Place the remaining ¼ cup broth in another saucepan. Add the remaining ingredients, except for ¼ cup of the green onions. Mix well and cook over medium heat for 20 minutes, stirring occasionally.

Mix the ¼ cup green onions into the cooked couscous and serve the tomato sauce over the couscous.

Quick Tip

Cut tomatoes with sharp scissors while still in the can.

DAIRY REPLACERS

All plant-based products

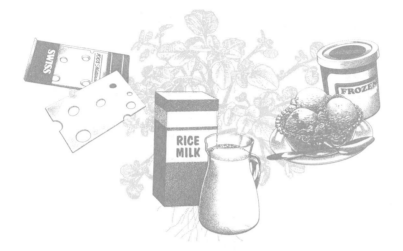

What am I going to put on my cereal if you won't let me have milk? The idea of drinking the milk of another animal is rather offensive. Would you drink dog milk? horse milk? monkey milk? Of course not. You had to make quite an adjustment as a child when your mother told you to "drink your milk for strong bones."

You can easily adjust to tasty substitutes for dairy products. You probably have your cereal right now with a sweetener like sugar or honey and fruit. You'll get the same flavors by replacing cow's milk with fruit juice. On cereal, juice provides moisture and sweetness, as well as a characteristic fruit flavor. If you want something creamy and white on your cereal try almond or cashew milk. Rice milk is low-fat and even healthier. Soy milk is often strong and tastes better when diluted with water.

The demand for dairy substitutes made of soy products has led to products that taste so much like the original your family will be fooled at the dinner table. There is soy cheese, soy yogurt, and soy ice cream. Most of them are very high in fat, but a few manufacturers are now making low-fat, high-protein varieties. These richer, plant-based substitutes should all be used sparingly (see the canned and packaged product list on page 286).

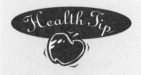

Powerful antioxidants, like beta carotene and vitamin C, that scavenge cell-damanging free radicals, are only found in plant foods. Dairy and meats are completely deficient in these cancer- and heart disease-fighting food components.

Fastest Dinner in the West

Servings: 2
Preparation Time:
5 minutes
Cooking Time:
10 minutes

8 ounces uncooked pasta of your choice
1 14.5-ounce can stewed tomatoes

½ cup medium salsa
½ cup mild salsa

Put a large pot of water on to boil. Drop the pasta into boiling water and cook according to the package directions. Drain and rinse.

Combine the remaining ingredients in a saucepan and cook until heated through, about 3 minutes. Combine the pasta with the sauce and serve at once.

Ravioli with Quick Marinara Sauce

Servings: 2 to 3
Preparation Time:
15 minutes
Cooking Time:
15 minutes

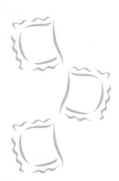

1 13-ounce package frozen Soy Boy Ravioli
¼ cup water
½ cup finely chopped onion
1 teaspoon minced fresh garlic

1 28-ounce can crushed tomatoes
2 teaspoons Italian seasoning blend
several twists of freshly ground black pepper

Put a large pot of water on to boil. When the water boils, drop in the ravioli and cook according to the package directions.

Meanwhile, place the ¼ cup water, onion, and garlic in a medium saucepan. Cook, stirring occasionally, for 3 minutes. Add the tomatoes, Italian seasoning, and pepper. Cook over low heat for 12 minutes, stirring occasionally.

Drain the ravioli and top with sauce.

Recipe Hint: *Soy Boy Ravioli is made by Northern Soy, Inc. It is an excellent nondairy ravioli. To stretch this sauce to cover two packages of ravioli, add 1 26-ounce jar of fat-free marinara sauce to the above recipe. This is a popular dish for most children. You can find other vegetable-filled ravioli in some natural food stores.*

Rotini and Greens

8 ounces uncooked rotini or other spiral pasta
2 tablespoons soy sauce
2 tablespoons sherry
2 tablespoons water
1 tablespoon lemon juice
1 tablespoon honey
1 teaspoon cornstarch
1 large Maui or Vidalia onion, sliced and separated into rings
¼ cup water
1 10-ounce package mixed salad greens

Servings: 4
Preparation Time:
10 minutes
Cooking Time:
10 minutes

Put a large pot of water on to boil. Drop the pasta into boiling water and cook according to the package directions. Drain and rinse.

Meanwhile, combine the soy sauce, sherry, 2 tablespoons water, the lemon juice, honey, and cornstarch in a bowl. Set aside.

Place the onion and ¼ cup water in a nonstick frying pan. Cook, stirring occasionally, for 5 minutes. Stir in the sauce mixture. Cook and stir until thickened. Remove from heat and add the pasta. Toss until well coated.

Place the greens in a large bowl. Add the pasta mixture and toss to mix. Serve at once.

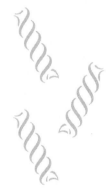

Oriental Soba Noodles

Servings: 4
Preparation Time:
15 minutes
Cooking Time:
10 minutes

8 ounces uncooked buckwheat
   soba noodles
1 cup vegetable broth
1 cup chopped green onions
2 cups sliced fresh shiitake
   mushrooms
1 red bell pepper, sliced into thin
   strips

½ teaspoon minced fresh garlic
¼ teaspoon crushed red pepper
2 cups sliced napa cabbage
1 6.5-ounce package Smoked
   Tofu, diced
2 tablespoons soy sauce
1 tablespoon mirin
1 tablespoon cornstarch

Put a large pot of water on to boil. Drop the soba noodles into boiling water and cook according to the package directions. Drain and rinse.

Meanwhile, place ½ cup of the broth in a large nonstick frying pan. Add the green onions, mushrooms, bell pepper, garlic, and crushed red pepper. Cook, stirring frequently, for 4 minutes. Add the cabbage and tofu. Cook for another 3 minutes. Combine the remaining ingredients with the rest of the vegetable broth and mix well. Stir into the vegetable mixture and cook and stir until thickened. Stir in the cooked noodles. Cook until heated through. Serve at once.

Recipe Hint: Smoked Tofu is made by Wildwood Natural Foods. It is sold in most natural food stores. If unavailable, use 1½ cups diced firm tofu or seitan in its place.

Pad Thai

8 ounces uncooked rice noodles
3 tablespoons soy sauce
2 tablespoons rice vinegar
2 tablespoons lime juice
1 tablespoon ketchup
2 teaspoons sugar
¼ teaspoon crushed red pepper
⅓ cup water
4 green onions, chopped

½ teaspoon minced fresh garlic
1 6.5-ounce package Smoked Tofu, thinly sliced
2 cups mung bean sprouts
½ cup shredded carrot
¼ cup chopped cilantro
2 tablespoons chopped peanuts (optional)

Servings: 4
Preparation Time: 15 minutes
Cooking Time: 10 minutes

Place the noodles in a bowl and cover with hot water. Soak for 10 minutes. Drain.

Combine the soy sauce, rice vinegar, lime juice, ketchup, sugar, and red pepper in a bowl. Mix well and set aside.

Place the water in a large nonstick frying pan. Add the green onions and garlic. Cook, stirring frequently, for 3 minutes. Add the tofu, bean sprouts, and noodles. Cook and stir for 2 minutes. Add the sauce mixture. Cook and stir for another 3 to 4 minutes until heated through. Transfer to a serving platter. Sprinkle with carrot, cilantro, and peanuts, if desired. Serve at once.

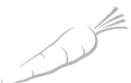

Recipe Hint: *Rice noodles can be found in most Asian markets. Made from rice and water, they are also called cellophane noodles. They do not need cooking; just soak in hot water to soften.*

ANIMAL PRODUCT
SUBSTITUTES

Egg Replacer
Agar-Agar
Guar Gum
Emes Kosher Gelatin
Soy Milk
Rice Milk

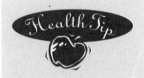

Infectious diseases are one important reason to avoid animal foods. Viruses, parasites, and bacteria cross species lines, easily transmitting diseases from cows, chickens, pigs, and fish to people.

*S*ubstitutes will eliminate the fat, cholesterol, and animal protein that animal products bring to the table. Egg Replacer (Ener-G Foods) is a flour product used to bind ingredients in place of eggs. (The product does not resemble eggs in any way.) When using Egg Replacer, be sure to beat the mixture in the water until it becomes frothy. Guar gum is used for thickening salad dressings instead of oil. It is stirred into the dressing and thickens in one hour without heating. Agar-agar and Emes Kosher Gelatin are used when a recipe such as molded salad calls for gelatin.

Rice and soy milk are used when you would use cow's milk in a recipe. They work well to make "cream" soups and stews. Textured vegetable protein and seitan (wheat protein) are used to make fake meats, poultry, and fish. Lunch meats, burgers, hot dogs, and cheeses made of soy and grain products can be used in recipes as meat substitutes. See the list of canned and packaged products on page 286 for some great substitution ideas.

Creamy Broccoli Pasta

8 ounces uncooked pasta of your choice
½ cup water
2 leeks, thinly sliced
2 cups small broccoli florets

1 cup soy or rice milk
2 teaspoons cornstarch
2 teaspoons chopped fresh basil
⅛ teaspoon Tabasco sauce

Servings: 4
Preparation Time:
10 minutes
Cooking Time:
10 minutes

Put a large pot of water on to boil. Drop in the pasta and cook according to the package directions. Drain and rinse.

Meanwhile, place the water, leeks, and broccoli in a saucepan. Cook, stirring frequently, for 8 minutes. Combine the remaining ingredients in a bowl. Add to the vegetable mixture and cook and stir until thickened. Serve over the pasta.

Pasta Jumble

⅓ cup water
1 onion, chopped
½ cup celery, chopped
½ teaspoon minced fresh garlic
1 28-ounce can chopped tomatoes
1 15-ounce can kidney beans, drained and rinsed
freshly ground black pepper to taste

½ pound uncooked spiral pasta
3 medium tomatoes, chopped
2 tablespoons chopped canned green chilies
2 leaves Swiss chard (stalks removed), sliced in ¼-inch pieces
dash or two of Tabasco sauce

Servings: 6
Preparation Time:
15 minutes
Cooking Time:
20 minutes

Place the water, onion, celery, and garlic in a large saucepan. Cook, stirring occasionally, for 5 minutes. Add the canned tomatoes and beans. Cook over low heat for 15 minutes. Season with the pepper.

Meanwhile, cook the spiral pasta in boiling water for 8 to 10 minutes, until just tender. Drain and add to the bean and tomato mixture. Add the fresh tomatoes, green chilies, Swiss chard, and Tabasco sauce. Cook until heated through.

Vegetable Pasta

Servings: 6 to 8
Preparation Time:
15 minutes
Cooking Time:
15 minutes

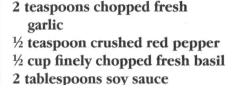

**2 teaspoons chopped fresh
    garlic**
½ teaspoon crushed red pepper
½ cup finely chopped fresh basil
2 tablespoons soy sauce

**1 pound uncooked vegetable
    spiral pasta**
**2 cups frozen chopped hash
    brown potatoes**
4 cups frozen mixed vegetables

Place the garlic, crushed red pepper, basil, and soy sauce in a small saucepan. Set aside. Bring 6 quarts of water to a boil in a large pot and cook the spiral pasta for 5 minutes; then add the potatoes and mixed vegetables and cook an additional 5 minutes. Drain the pasta and vegetables, saving some of the cooking water. Add 1 cup of the cooking water to the garlic-basil mixture and heat it in the saucepan. Pour the heated mixture into the pasta and vegetables. Mix all ingredients together, adding reserved cooking water as needed for moisture.

Artichoke Pasta Sauce

Servings: 6
Preparation Time:
10 minutes
Cooking Time:
20 minutes

½ cup water
1 onion, chopped
1 green bell pepper, chopped
1½ teaspoons minced fresh garlic
**1 16-ounce can water-packed
    artichoke hearts, drained**

**⅛ cup sliced black olives
    (optional)**
**2 15-ounce cans fat-free pasta
    sauce**
1 teaspoon dill weed

Place the water in a saucepan with the onion, bell pepper, and garlic. Cook, stirring frequently, until tender, about 10 minutes. Add the remaining ingredients and bring to a boil. Reduce heat, cover, and simmer over low heat for 10 minutes.

Recipe Hint: Try this sauce over angel hair pasta. Put the water on to boil when you start this recipe and drop the pasta in when you cover the sauce for the final cooking.

Oriental Pasta

1 teaspoon minced fresh garlic
1 teaspoon grated fresh
  gingerroot
⅛ to ¼ teaspoon crushed red
  pepper
1 cup shredded carrot
2 cups broccoli florets
½ cup water

¼ cup soy sauce
½ pound sliced fresh mushrooms
1 bunch green onions cut into
  1-inch pieces
½ pound uncooked udon or soba
  noodles
1 tablespoon cornstarch mixed in
  2 tablespoons cold water

Servings: 4
Preparation Time:
15 minutes
Cooking Time:
15 minutes

Place the garlic, ginger, red pepper, carrot, and broccoli in a wok or large pan with the ½ cup water and 2 tablespoons of the soy sauce. Cook and stir for 5 minutes. Add the mushrooms and green onions. Cook, covered, for about 5 minutes.

Meanwhile, prepare the pasta according to the package directions. Drain. Toss with the remaining 2 tablespoons soy sauce.

Add the cornstarch mixture to the vegetable mixture, cook, and stir until thickened. Add to the pasta. Mix well.

Recipe Hint: *Add some baby corn, snow peas, and/or chopped leafy greens when you add the mushrooms for more variety. Buy shredded carrot and chopped broccoli in bags and use presliced mushrooms to save time.*

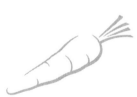

Meaty Mushroom Stroganoff

Servings: 6
Preparation Time:
15 minutes
Cooking Time:
30 minutes

1 pound uncooked fettuccine
⅓ cup water
1 large onion, chopped
1 pound sliced fresh mushrooms
1 8-ounce package Beyond Roast
   Beef, thawed and sliced
dash of cayenne pepper

2 tablespoons white wine
2 tablespoons soy sauce
1 cup soy milk
1 cup vegetable broth
2 tablespoons cornstarch mixed
   in ¼ cup cold water

Put a large pot of water on to boil. Drop the fettuccine into boiling water and cook according to the package directions. Drain and rinse.

Meanwhile, place the water and onion in a large nonstick frying pan and cook for 2 to 3 minutes. Add the mushrooms and cook until they are slightly limp. Add the remaining ingredients, except for the cornstarch mixture. Mix. Cover and cook over low heat for 20 minutes, stirring occasionally. Add the cornstarch mixture to the pan, cook, and stir until thickened.

Serve over the fettuccine.

Recipe Hint: *Beyond Roast Beef is made by Ivy Foods in Salt Lake City. It is sold frozen in most natural food stores. Savory Seitan by Lightlife Foods in Greenfield, Massachusetts, is another delicious gluten product that may be used in this recipe. These products are made from wheat gluten and taste very similar to meat. They are often referred to as "meat from wheat."*

PASTA—FAST & EASY

Pasta

Most dry pastas cook in eight to ten minutes. Smaller pastas, such as orzo, cook even faster (five minutes). Couscous is a pasta that can be prepared by pouring boiling water over it and letting it sit for five minutes. Fresh pastas cook in two to four minutes.

To cook pasta, bring a large pot of water to a boil. Drop the pasta into the boiling water a little at a time so you don't stop the boiling. Stir to separate, then cook uncovered at a rolling boil until tender. Check the pasta frequently toward the end of the cooking time so that it doesn't get too soft. Test by biting into the pasta. It should be firm but not overcooked. If you are going to serve it hot with a sauce, drain, but do not rinse. Rinsing removes the starch on the pasta that helps the sauce stick to it. To serve cold in salads, drain and rinse in cold water. Leftover pasta can be frozen. Pasta reheats easily in a microwave.

The best way to cook pasta is in a large stainless steel pot with a removable liner with holes in it. When the pasta is finished cooking, just lift the liner out of the boiling water, shake, and pour the pasta into a bowl. This avoids the old awkward and dangerous method of pouring a heavy pot of boiling water and pasta noodles into a colander.

Multiple sclerosis is rare where the diet is low in animal fats, and high in plant foods, such as traditional pasta-eating Italians and rice-eating Japanese. A low-fat diet is also the best treatment for MS.

Spicy Mongolian Noodles

Servings: 4
Preparation Time:
15 minutes
Cooking Time:
10 minutes

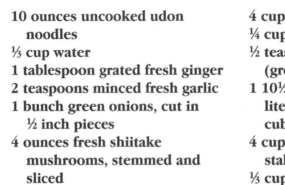

10 ounces uncooked udon
  noodles
⅓ cup water
1 tablespoon grated fresh ginger
2 teaspoons minced fresh garlic
1 bunch green onions, cut in
  ½ inch pieces
4 ounces fresh shiitake
  mushrooms, stemmed and
  sliced

4 cups vegetable broth
¼ cup soy sauce
½ teaspoon Sambal Oelek
  (ground fresh chili paste)
1 10½-ounce package extra firm
  lite silken tofu, cut into
  cubes
4 cups sliced bok choy greens,
  stalks removed
⅓ cup chopped cilantro

Bring a large pot of water to a boil. Add the noodles and cook until tender, 8 to 10 minutes. Drain and set aside.

Meanwhile, place the ⅓ cup water, ginger and garlic in a large soup pot. Cook, stirring, for 2 minutes. Add the onions and mushrooms and cook for 3 minutes. Add the broth, soy sauce and chili paste. Cover and bring to a boil. Add the tofu and bok choy and cook for 2 minutes. Turn off the heat and add the cooked noodles and cilantro. Stir to mix. Serve at once.

Recipe Hint: *To save time, shred the bok choy in a food processor. If you can't find shiitake mushrooms, use cremini or oyster mushrooms.*

Pasta with Chili Sauce

1 pound uncooked pasta of your
choice
1 15-ounce can fat-free vegetarian
chili
1 15-ounce can tomato sauce

1 14.5-ounce can stewed
tomatoes
½ cup water
1 onion, finely chopped

Servings: 4
Preparation Time:
5 minutes
Cooking Time:
10 minutes

Put a large pot of water on to boil. Drop the pasta into boiling water and cook according to the package directions.

Place the chili, tomato sauce, stewed tomatoes, and water in a saucepan. Cook, stirring occasionally, for 5 minutes.

Drain the pasta and place in a bowl. Pour the sauce over the pasta and serve topped with the chopped onion. This is also good over brown rice or potatoes.

Fresh Basil and Pepper Pasta

1 pound uncooked vegetable
curly pasta
⅓ cup water
1 bunch green onions, chopped
1 15-ounce can garbanzo beans,
drained and rinsed

1 10-ounce jar roasted red
peppers, chopped
⅓ cup chopped fresh basil leaves
1 tablespoon drained capers
freshly ground black pepper to
taste

Servings: 4
Preparation Time:
15 minutes
Cooking Time:
10 minutes

Put a large pot of water on to boil. Drop the pasta into boiling water and cook according to the package directions.

Meanwhile, place the water in a sauce pot with the green onions. Cook for 2 minutes, then add the remaining ingredients. Cook, stirring frequently, for 5 minutes.

Drain the pasta and place in a bowl. Pour the sauce over and mix well. Serve at once.

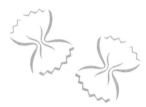

Quick Tip

Stack the basil leaves in piles and cut with sharp knife.

Summer Fettuccine

Servings: 8
Preparation Time:
15 minutes
Cooking Time:
20 minutes

1 pound fettuccine or other pasta
½ cup water
½ teaspoon minced fresh garlic
1 small onion, cut in wedges
2 large tomatoes, chopped
2 yellow summer squash, thinly
  sliced
1 cup cut fresh green beans

1 cup corn
¼ cup finely chopped fresh
  basil
2 tablespoons chopped fresh
  parsley
1 6-ounce can tomato paste
freshly ground black pepper to
  taste

Bring a large pot of water to a boil. Add the pasta and cook according to package directions.

Place the water in a large saucepan. Add the garlic and onion and cook for 2 minutes. Add the tomatoes, squash, green beans, and corn. Cook, stirring frequently, for 5 minutes.

Add the basil, parsley, and tomato paste. Cook over low heat, stirring occasionally, for about 15 minutes, or until vegetables are tender. Season to taste with pepper.

Drain the pasta in a large bowl. Spoon the sauce over the pasta and serve immediately.

Recipe Hint: *1 cup of sliced mushrooms may be substituted for the corn, and zucchini may be substituted for the summer squash. Try this with gnocchi instead of pasta.*

Mustardy Pasta

1 pound uncooked linguine or spaghetti

2 cups small cauliflower florets

2 cups small broccoli florets

¼ cup water

½ cup thinly sliced leeks

1 teaspoon minced fresh garlic

1 tomato, chopped

2 tablespoons snipped fresh parsley

2 tablespoons Dijon-style mustard

1 tablespoon balsamic vinegar

several twists of freshly ground black pepper

soy parmesan cheese (optional)

Servings: 6 to 8
Preparation Time:
15 minutes
Cooking Time:
10 to 12 minutes

Put a large pot of water on to boil. Drop the pasta into boiling water and cook according to the package directions. Add the cauliflower and broccoli during the last 3 minutes of cooking time.

Meanwhile, place the water in a small nonstick saucepan. Add the leeks and garlic. Cook, stirring occasionally, for 2 minutes. Add the tomato, parsley, mustard, vinegar, and pepper. Cook for another 3 minutes, stirring occasionally.

Drain the pasta and vegetables. Place in a bowl. Add the tomato mixture and toss well to mix. Sprinkle with some soy parmesan cheese, if desired. Serve at once.

BARBECUES & PICNICS

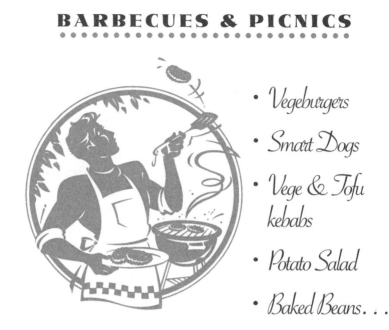

• *Vegeburgers*

• *Smart Dogs*

• *Vege & Tofu kebabs*

• *Potato Salad*

• *Baked Beans...*

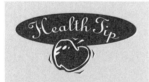

Some sunshine is necessary for good health. Your best source of vitamin D is sunlight which converts plant sterols to the active vitamin in your skin. Milk is naturally deficient in vitamin D, and only contains this fat-soluble vitamin if added during manufacturing.

*S*ummertime barbecues are an American tradition that healthy vegetarians don't have to give up. You can grill vegetarian hot dogs made from nonfat soy products and gluten and hamburgers made from nonfat soy products, gluten, potatoes, legumes, and/or grain products (see recipe on page 203 and the list of canned and packaged products on page 286). Place between whole wheat buns and use all your favorite condiments: mustard, ketchup, pickle relish, onions, lettuce, and tomatoes. Shish kebabs are made with marinated vegetables and grilled. Roast corn on the cob and foil-and-parchment-paper wrapped potatoes and vegetables. Bring a healthy potato salad, baked beans, or green salad with fat-free dressing (see recipes on pages 48–52). If you don't mention it, friends and family who still insist on burning the cow on a sunny holiday afternoon won't even notice you're eating something different.

Grilling over charcoal or gas flames? Combustion of fats from the foods produces cancer-causing substances. Fortunately, with low-fat foods you will avoid the drippings that can cause such reactions. Wood smoke and charcoal also contain substances that may cause cancer. Gas flame grills are the cleanest; however, you may feel that too much is sacrificed by avoiding the familiar flavors left by the burning wood or charcoal.

Creamy Spinach Pasta

10 ounces dried spinach fettuccine
1 6-ounce bag triple-washed baby spinach leaves
1 cup fresh basil leaves
½ teaspoon fresh minced garlic

1 cup soft lite silken tofu
dash salt
⅔ cup vegetable broth
1½ cups halved cherry tomatoes
freshly ground black pepper to taste

Servings: 4 to 6
Preparation Time:
15 minutes
Cooking Time:
10 minutes

Bring a large pot of water to a boil. Add the pasta and cook according to package directions. Just before the pasta is done, add the spinach and cook until wilted, 30 to 45 seconds.

Meanwhile, place the basil and garlic in a food processor and process just until chopped. Add the tofu and the salt. Process until smooth. Place in a saucepan with the vegetable broth and heat gently—do not boil.

Drain the fettuccine and spinach. Place in a serving bowl, pour the tofu mixture over the pasta and toss well to mix. Sprinkle the cherry tomatoes over the pasta and season with pepper.

Recipe Hint: *To make this dish a little spicier, add a dash or two of Tabasco sauce to the tofu mixture. If you are a real spinach lover, use two bags of the baby spinach leaves instead of one.*

Bresson's Noodles and Beans

Servings: 8
Preparation Time:
15 minutes
Cooking Time:
20 minutes

1 12-ounce package spiral
  pasta
⅓ cup water
1 onion, chopped
1 green bell pepper, chopped
1 cup sliced fresh mushrooms
1 stalk celery, sliced

1 small zucchini, chopped
1 15-ounce can black beans,
  drained and rinsed
1 15-ounce can garbanzo beans,
  drained and rinsed
1 14.5-ounce can stewed
  tomatoes

Put a large pot of water on to boil. Drop the pasta into boiling water and cook according to the package directions. Drain.

Meanwhile, place the water in a large sauce pot. Add the onion, bell pepper, mushrooms, celery, and zucchini. Cook, stirring frequently, for 5 minutes. Add the remaining ingredients and the pasta. Mix well and simmer over low heat for 15 minutes.

Recipe Hint: To change the flavor of this dish, use Italian-style, Mexican-style, or Cajun-style stewed tomatoes. This recipe freezes well.

Pasta Primavera

½ cup water
1 tablespoon soy sauce
1 cup sliced fresh mushrooms
1 cup broccoli florets
2 green onions, chopped
1 teaspoon minced fresh
  garlic
8 ounces uncooked linguine or
  spaghetti
2 cups snow pea pods

6 asparagus spears, cut into
  1½-inch pieces
1 red bell pepper, cut into thin
  strips
½ cup soy or rice milk
1 teaspoon slivered fresh basil
several twists of freshly ground
  black pepper
¼ cup soy parmesan cheese
  (optional)

Servings: 4
Preparation Time:
15 minutes
Cooking Time:
15 minutes

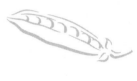

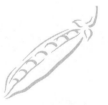

Put a large pot of water on to boil before starting to cook the vegetables.

Place the water and soy sauce in a large frying pan. Add the mushrooms, broccoli, green onions, and garlic. Cook, stirring frequently, for 5 minutes.

Drop the pasta into boiling water.

Add the snow peas, asparagus, and bell pepper to the vegetables. Cook for another 5 minutes. Add the milk, basil, and pepper. Cook, stirring occasionally, for another 5 minutes.

Drain the pasta. Ladle the vegetables over the pasta and top with the soy parmesan cheese, if desired.

Quick Tip

For perfect pasta every time, bring the water to a boil. Add the pasta a little at a time so that the water does not stop boiling and the pasta doesn't stick together.

DINING OUT
MCDOUGALL–STYLE

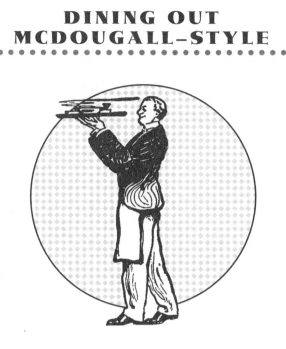

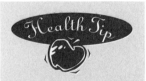

People fail to find healthy restaurant meals when they don't commit to eat right before they look at the menu. When faced with less than ideal food selections, choose white rice and white bread over animal products and greasy foods.

We can find a healthy, great-tasting meal for ourselves in eight out of ten restaurants. For breakfast, John orders a whole grain cold cereal with fruit juice or hot oatmeal, hash brown potatoes cooked without grease and topped with salsa or ketchup, whole wheat toast and jelly, fresh fruit, and herbal tea. For lunch and dinner, we look for a vegetarian restaurant and stay away from the eggs, cheese, and oil on their menu. Chinese, Thai, and Japanese restaurants can easily make an oil-free, animal-free topping to go over rice (usually white rice). Indian restaurants have a tradition of vegetarian cooking—tell the waiter to "hold the ghee" (clarified butter). Chefs at most fine dining establishments consider cooking you a pure vegetarian dish with no oil to be a welcome challenge—if you give them notice.

Fast meals can be had at salad bars—just leave out the selections with mayonnaise and olive oil. Many Mexican restaurants can put together a burrito or tostada made with oil-free pinto or black beans, lettuce, tomatoes, and salsa. Pizza without the cheese is almost perfect, except for the oil in the crust and the white flour. Top with generous amounts of tomato sauce and vegetables. Jusk ask. You'll be surprised how happy most restaurants are to have your business.

Mushroom Stroganoff

6 tablespoons white wine
1 onion, chopped
1 pound sliced fresh mushrooms
2 tablespoons soy sauce
1 10-ounce package lite silken
  tofu

1 tablespoon lemon juice
½ teaspoon Worcestershire
  sauce
freshly ground black pepper to
  taste

Servings: 4
Preparation Time:
10 minutes
Cooking Time:
8 minutes

Place 3 tablespoons of the wine in a large frying pan. Add the onion and cook, stirring occasionally, for 3 minutes. Add the mushrooms, 2 tablespoons of the wine, and the soy sauce. Cook, stirring frequently, for 5 minutes.

Meanwhile, place the tofu in a food processor with the remaining 1 tablespoon wine and the lemon juice. Process until smooth. Pour into the pan with the mushrooms and onions. Mix well. Add the remaining ingredients and stir until heated through.

Serve over pasta.

> **Recipe Hint:** *Put the water on to boil for the pasta when you start to cook the onions. When the water is boiling, drop the pasta in and it will be ready at about the same time as the stroganoff. To save time, buy presliced mushrooms.*

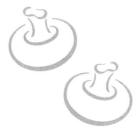

Mexican Pasta

Servings: 6
Preparation Time:
15 minutes
Cooking Time:
10 minutes

1 pound uncooked fettuccine
1 onion, chopped
1 green bell pepper, chopped
1 teaspoon minced fresh garlic
½ cup water
1 15-ounce can black beans,
   drained and rinsed
1 cup frozen corn kernels

1½ cups chopped tomatoes
1 4-ounce can diced green
   chilies
½ teaspoon oregano
½ teaspoon chili powder
1 tablespoon chopped fresh
   cilantro
1 lime (optional)

Cook the fettuccine according to the package directions. Drain and set aside. Meanwhile, place the onion, bell pepper, garlic, and water in a large pot. Cook, stirring frequently, for 4 minutes. Add the beans, corn, tomatoes, green chilies, oregano, and chili powder. Cook, stirring frequently, for 5 minutes. Add the cooked fettuccine and cilantro. Cook until heated through, about 1 minute. Cut the lime in half and squeeze the juice over the pasta before serving, if desired.

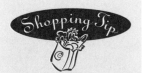

Shopping Tip

Make a list for each store you plan to shop at: the supermarket and the natural food store. Group items according to the floor plan of the store to prevent duplication of steps. Start with the first section you come to, then methodically imagine a walk through the store.

Mexican Seitan Pasta

1 onion, chopped
1 cup water
8 ounces beef-flavored seitan, chopped
2 14.5-ounce cans Mexican-style stewed tomatoes

1 cup uncooked pasta (wagon wheels, macaroni, small shapes: trees, leaves, etc.)

Servings: 4 to 6
Preparation Time: 5 minutes
Cooking Time: 25 minutes

Place the onion in a medium pot with ⅓ cup of the water. Cook and stir for 1 minute. Add the seitan. Cook, stirring frequently, for 4 minutes. Add the tomatoes and remaining water. Bring to a boil. Add the pasta. Cover and cook over low heat, stirring occasionally, for 20 minutes, until the pasta is tender.

Recipe Hint: *There are many seitan products on the market (see the canned and packaged products list on page 286).*

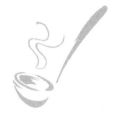

Bow Ties with Bean Sauce

Servings: 4 to 6
Preparation Time:
15 minutes
Cooking Time:
10 minutes

1 pound uncooked bow tie
  pasta
½ cup vegetable broth
½ teaspoon minced fresh
  garlic
1 10-ounce bag washed spinach,
  chopped

1 15-ounce can cannellini beans,
  drained and rinsed
1 15-ounce can red beans,
  drained and rinsed
1 tablespoon soy parmesan
  cheese
¼ teaspoon red pepper flakes

Cook the pasta according to the package directions. Drain well.

Meanwhile, place the vegetable broth in a large saucepan. Add the garlic and cook for 2 minutes. Add the spinach and stir frequently until it has wilted, about 3 minutes. Add the remaining ingredients. Mix well and cook for another 5 minutes.

Toss the bean mixture with the hot pasta. Serve at once.

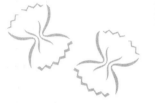

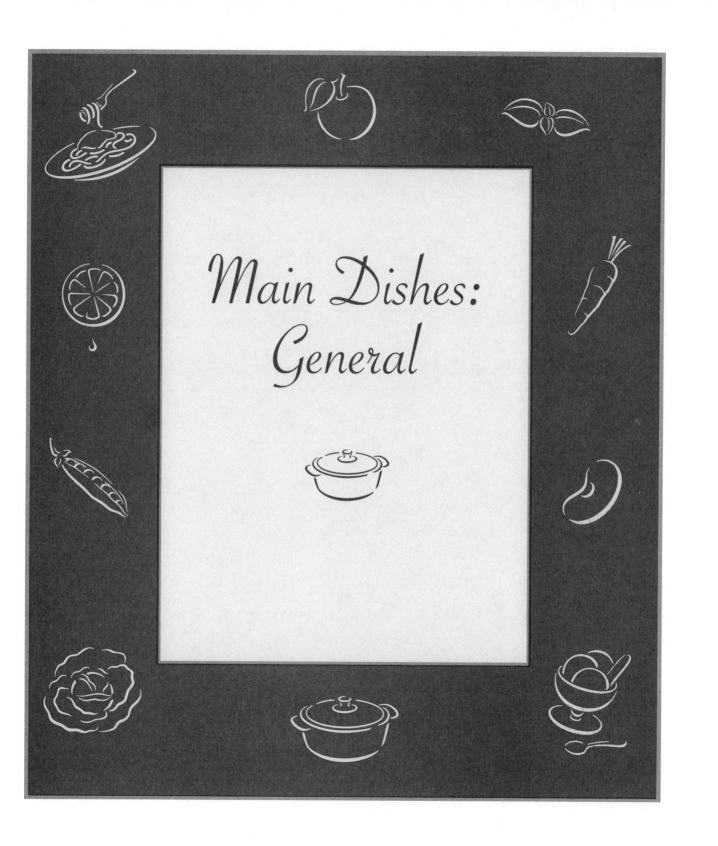

Main Dishes: General

Haystacks

8 cups fat-free baked tortilla
  chips
1 recipe Fast Refried Beans
  (page 124)

¾ cup chopped green onions
2 cups salsa

1 4-ounce can diced green chilies
1 4-ounce can chopped ripe
  olives (optional)
1 cup chopped tomatoes

Servings: 8
Preparation Time:
15 minutes
Cooking Time:
10 minutes

Place all ingredients in separate bowls. To assemble, layer ingredients over the chips in the order given. Eat with your fingers, or use a fork if you must.

Vegetable Burritos

⅓ cup water
1 onion, chopped
1 red bell pepper, chopped
½ pound sliced mushrooms
2 zucchini, chopped

1 10-ounce can Ro-tel chopped
  tomatoes and green
  chilies
2 cups chopped fresh spinach
6 to 8 whole wheat tortillas

Servings: 6 to 8
Preparation Time:
15 minutes
Cooking Time:
16 minutes

Place the water in a large frying pan. Add the onion and bell pepper. Cook, stirring occasionally, for 5 minutes. Add the mushrooms and zucchini and cook for 5 minutes longer. Stir in the tomatoes and cook for another 5 minutes. Add the spinach and stir until wilted, about 1 minute.

Place a line of the vegetable mixture down the center of a tortilla, roll up, and eat.

Recipe Hint: *Buy sliced mushrooms in the supermarket. Use a food processor to chop the onion, bell pepper, and zucchini. This may also be used as a stuffing for pita bread.*

INSTANT CUP MEALS

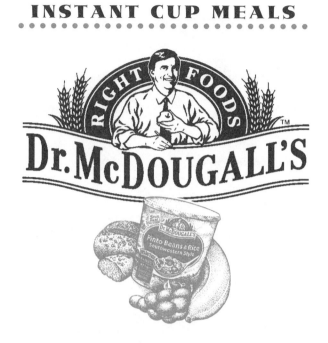

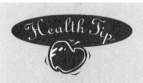
*C*onvenience is almost as important to most people as healthfulness when choosing foods these days. Dehydrated meals in a cup are a four-step (thirty-second) process: (1) boil water, (2) pour water into cup, (3) stir, and (4) cover and wait five minutes. You can have oatmeal for breakfast, split pea soup for lunch, rice and pasta pilaf for dinner, and a rice pudding for dessert. Those with a heartier appetite can add a microwaved baked potato or a green salad to lunch and dinner or have two cups. The soups and dinners make a great topping for rice, pasta, or a baked potato.

There are many manufacturers of instant cup meals and a wide range of quality. Begin by reading the label; check for animal products (milk, butter powder, whey, chicken, eggs, etc.), added oil, and excessive salt. Some companies skimp on ingredients which leaves you with an uninteresting and sometimes inedible meal.

Dr. McDougall's Right Foods are lower in sodium than most instant cup meals (480 mg/cup or less) and use only the best quality, mineral-rich, natural sea salt. The finest ingredients from around the world are combined to bring you one of the few prepared foods that doesn't have that packaged food flavor. Find them in your grocery and natural food store or call (800) 367-3844 to order by mail.

Tostadas

6 to 8 soft corn tortillas
2 15-ounce cans nonfat refried
  beans
1½ teaspoons chili powder
½ teaspoon ground cumin

¼ teaspoon garlic powder
2 tomatoes, chopped
1 bunch green onions, chopped
1 cup shredded lettuce
1 cup fresh salsa

Servings: 6 to 8
Preparation Time:
15 minutes
Cooking Time:
10 minutes

Preheat the oven to 350 degrees.

Place the corn tortillas on a nonstick baking sheet and bake until crispy, about 10 minutes.

Meanwhile, combine the beans with the chili powder, cumin, and garlic powder in a small saucepan. Cook over low heat until heated through, about 10 minutes.

Spread the bean mixture over crisp tortillas and top with the tomatoes, green onions, lettuce, and salsa.

Soft Black Bean Tostadas

3 15-ounce cans black beans,
  undrained
2 teaspoons chili powder
1 teaspoon ground cumin
dash or two of Tabasco sauce

6 soft corn tortillas
2 tomatoes, chopped
1½ cups shredded leaf lettuce
1 cup fresh salsa

Servings: 6
Preparation Time:
10 minutes
Cooking Time:
10 minutes

Place the beans in a saucepan with the chili powder, cumin, and Tabasco sauce. Cook over low heat until heated through, about 10 minutes. Place about ½ cup of beans on a plate. Place 1 corn tortilla over the beans and flatten slightly. Cover the tortilla with more beans, then layer on the remaining ingredients in the order listed. Repeat with the remaining tortillas.

Southwest Vegetable Burritos

Servings: 6
Preparation Time:
15 minutes
Cooking Time:
10 minutes

½ cup water
1 bunch green onions, chopped
1 green bell pepper, sliced into strips
1 red bell pepper, sliced into strips
1 cup sliced fresh mushrooms
1 zucchini, cut lengthwise in quarters, then sliced

1 cup frozen corn kernels, thawed
1 tablespoon cornstarch
1½ cups salsa
12 cherry tomatoes, cut in half
¼ cup chopped fresh cilantro
6 large whole wheat tortillas

Place the water in a large nonstick frying pan. Add the green onions, bell peppers, mushrooms, and zucchini. Cook, stirring occasionally, for 5 minutes. Add the corn and cook for another 2 to 3 minutes.

Mix the cornstarch into the salsa and add to the vegetables. Cook, stirring until thickened. Add the tomatoes and cook for 1 minute longer. Stir in the cilantro and remove from heat.

To serve, place a line of the vegetable mixture down the center of a tortilla and top with more salsa, if desired. Roll up and eat.

Quick Tip

Mix leftover bean or vegetable dishes with bread or cracker crumbs, or oatmeal. Flatten the mixture into pancakes and layer between plastic wrap or parchment paper. Freeze. Brown on a nonstick griddle or bake in the oven; serve with gravy or sauce or top with an instant soup cup.

Vegetable Bean Enchiladas

⅓ cup water
½ cup chopped green bell pepper
½ cup chopped green onions
1 15-ounce can black beans, drained and rinsed
1 cup frozen corn kernels, thawed

1 tablespoon diced canned green chilies
2 teaspoons minced fresh garlic
2 teaspoons ground cumin
3 cups Enchilada Sauce (page 221)
10 to 12 corn tortillas

Servings: 4 to 6
Preparation Time:
15 minutes
Cooking Time:
30 minutes

Place the water, bell pepper, and green onions in a saucepan. Cook, stirring occasionally, for 5 minutes. Add the beans, corn, chilies, garlic, and cumin. Mix well.

Preheat the oven to 375 degrees.

Pour 1 cup of the enchilada sauce in the bottom of a baking dish.

Wrap the tortillas in a cloth and heat on high in the microwave for 1 minute. Spoon about ¼ cup of the bean mixture on each and roll up. Lay seam side down in the baking dish. Pour the remaining sauce over the top. Bake for 15 to 20 minutes, or until bubbly. Remove from the oven and serve at once.

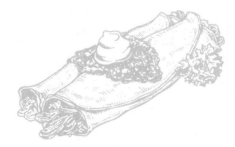

EXERCISE FOR HEALTH & FITNESS

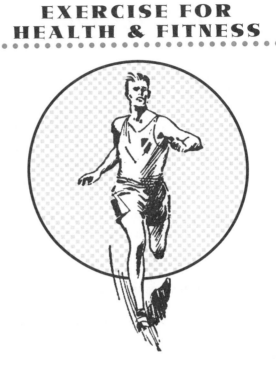

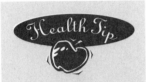

It is safer and more effective to add time to your exercise than to increase intensity. Add ten minutes to a thirty-minute session and burn 33 percent more calories.

You can lose weight and improve your health simply by changing your diet. But why not get really healthy and fit with daily exercise? At least thirty minutes done three to five days a week is best. Most important is to find an exercise program you enjoy so you will keep doing it. Walking is something almost anyone can do safely. More strenuous exercises will require conditioning and training. Consider joining a health club or hiring a personal certified exercise trainer to get professional help and get off to the right start.

With exercise you lose weight faster and put on attractive muscle. You reduce your risk of heart disease. Blood pressure and triglycerides go down, and "good" HDL cholesterol goes up. Exercise reduces stress and relieves minor anxiety and depression. Overall, studies show you will live longer if you make regular exercise a part of your life.

You certainly should change your diet before you start a serious exercise program, because this change will overnight reduce your risk of a heart attack, which may be brought on by overexertion. You may also want to see your doctor before you start, especially if you have had health problems in the past.

Potato Enchiladas

2 16-ounce jars Parrot Brand
  Enchilada Sauce
⅓ cup salsa
2 cups mashed potatoes (see hint)
8 to 10 whole wheat tortillas or
  soft corn tortillas

¾ cup chopped green onions
¾ cup frozen corn kernels,
  thawed
1 4-ounce can diced green
  chilies

*Servings: 4 to 6
Preparation Time:
10 minutes (need
mashed potatoes)
Cooking Time:
30 minutes*

Preheat the oven to 350 degrees.

Spread 1 cup of the sauce over the bottom of a covered casserole dish. Stir the salsa into the mashed potatoes and mix well. Spread a line of potatoes down the center of each tortilla; sprinkle on some green onions, corn, and green chilies. Roll up and place seam side down in the casserole. Repeat until all ingredients are used. Pour the remaining sauce over the tortillas, cover, and bake for 30 minutes.

__Recipe Hint:__ If you do not have leftover mashed potatoes, use instant mashed potatoes. Make them with all water or use water and soy or rice milk. Do not add butter or oil. We also make a soft potato mixture by cooking frozen chopped hash brown potatoes in water until soft. Use twice as many potatoes as water and cook for about 25 minutes. If you prefer to make your own enchilada sauce, there is an easy recipe on page 221.

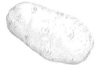
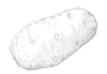

Spinach-Rice Enchiladas

Servings: 4 to 6
Preparation Time:
10 minutes
(need cooked rice)
Cooking Time:
35 minutes

¼ cup water
1 onion, chopped
1 6-ounce bag triple-washed baby
    spinach leaves
2 cups cooked brown rice

1 tablespoon soy sauce
1 teaspoon ground cumin
2 16-ounce jars Parrot Brand
    Enchilada Sauce
8 to 10 soft corn tortillas

Preheat the oven to 350 degrees.

Place the water and onion in a medium saucepan. Cook, stirring occasionally, until the onion softens slightly, about 3 minutes. Add the spinach and stir until it softens, about 2 minutes. Remove from heat. Add the rice, soy sauce, and cumin. Mix and set aside.

Spread 1 cup of the sauce over the bottom of a covered casserole dish. Spread a line of the spinach-rice mixture down the center of each tortilla. Roll up and place seam side down in the casserole. Repeat until all ingredients are used. Pour the remaining sauce over the tortillas, cover, and bake for 30 minutes.

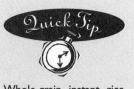

Quick Tip

Whole-grain instant rice and quick-cooking oatmeal are found on supermarket shelves and can be made in a fraction of the time as the original grain. Instant mashed potatoes (made without milk or eggs) are reconstituted in minutes with a little hot water.

Black Bean, Corn, and Rice Burritos

Servings: 12
Preparation Time:
15 minutes
(need cooked rice)
Cooking Time:
10 minutes

1½ cups salsa
1 15-ounce can black beans, drained and rinsed
1 11-ounce can corn, drained and rinsed
1 4-ounce can chopped green chilies
1 tomato, chopped

½ teaspoon minced fresh garlic
1 teaspoon chili powder
½ teaspoon ground cumin
2 cups cooked brown rice
12 fat-free flour tortillas
½ cup chopped green onions
¼ cup chopped cilantro

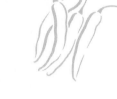

Place ½ cup of the salsa in a saucepan. Add the beans, corn, green chilies, tomato, garlic, chili powder, and cumin. Cook, stirring occasionally, for about 8 minutes. Stir in the rice and heat through.

Wrap the tortillas in a cloth and heat for 2 minutes in the microwave. Spread a line of the bean and rice mixture down the center of each tortilla, sprinkle on a few green onions and cilantro, then finish with some of the salsa. Roll up and eat.

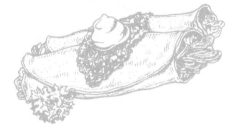

Mexican Lasagne

Servings: 8
Preparation Time:
10 minutes
Cooking Time:
35 minutes

1 small onion, chopped
1 cup sliced fresh mushrooms
⅓ cup water
2 14.5-ounce cans Mexican-style
  stewed tomatoes
2 15-ounce cans pinto beans,
  drained and rinsed

1 4-ounce can chopped green
  chilies
1 teaspoon chili powder
8 corn tortillas
1 bunch green onions, finely
  chopped

Preheat the oven to 350 degrees.

Place the onion and mushrooms in a medium saucepan with the water. Cook, stirring occasionally, for 2 minutes. Add the tomatoes, beans, chilies, and chili powder. Mix well and cook for 3 minutes.

Place 4 of the corn tortillas over the bottom of a nonstick 9 × 12-inch baking dish. Pour half of the bean mixture over the tortillas. Layer the remaining tortillas over the bean mixture, then pour the remaining bean mixture over the tortillas. Sprinkle the green onions over the top and bake for 30 minutes.

Recipe Hint: *You could sprinkle some grated soy cheese over the top of this casserole, if desired. Also, it may be made without the onions and mushrooms. Combine the tomatoes, beans, chilies, and chili powder in a bowl. Then just layer the tortillas as above and bake as directed.*

WHAT KIND OF A COOK ARE YOU?

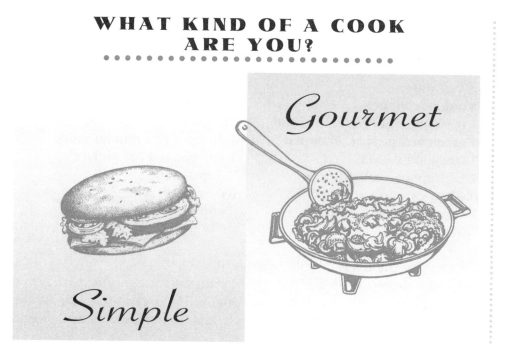

Gourmet

Simple

*A*re you the kind of cook who spends hours thinking about and preparing your meals? You can modify your gourmet recipes by leaving out the oils and animal products. There are over 1,700 recipes in the McDougall books. Many recipes are quite elaborate and take time. Most of the meals in our home are made in the style of this book—quick and easy, but still very tasty. For example, Mary will make a bowl of pasta with marinara sauce and serve it with a simple green salad. A soup meal in our home is a large pot of bean or vegetable soup served with a loaf of fresh bread.

If you're a simple cook, then vegetable foods are ideal for you. Bake a potato or two in the microwave. Boil a bag of precooked frozen vegetables. Top the potatoes with salsa, oil-free salad dressing, or an instant soup. Make a low-fat vegetable burger with a whole wheat bun and garnish with lettuce, tomatoes, onions, mustard, ketchup, and relish. Boil some pasta and top with a bottled marinara sauce. This entire book is dedicated to the cook who doesn't want to spend time in the kitchen but still wants great-tasting meals.

People often tell us that since changing their diets they enjoy cooking again. Many women comment on their husbands' newfound interest in shopping and cooking the meals. New foods offer new challenges and enjoyments.

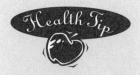

Health Tip

Greater variety of foods usually means greater calorie intake. For faster, greater weight loss make your meals simple and repetitious. A monotonous style of eating can be healthy, timesaving, and economical.

Tex-Mex Lasagne

Servings: 6
Preparation Time:
15 minutes
Cooking Time:
23 minutes

⅓ cup water
1 onion, chopped
1 teaspoon minced fresh garlic
1 green bell pepper, chopped
1 teaspoon cumin
1 tablespoon chili powder
dash of cayenne pepper
1 cup frozen corn kernels, thawed

1 15-ounce can pinto or kidney beans, drained and rinsed
1 8-ounce can tomato sauce
1 cup cooked brown rice (optional)
6 corn tortillas
1 cup tofu, mashed

Preheat the oven to 350 degrees.

Place the water in a large frying pan; add the onion, garlic, and bell pepper. Cook, stirring occasionally, for 3 minutes. Stir in the spices and mix well. Add the corn, beans, tomato sauce, and rice, if desired.

Place 3 of the tortillas in the bottom of a 2-quart casserole dish. Pour half of the bean mixture over the tortillas and spread half of the tofu over the beans. Repeat with the remaining ingredients. Bake for 20 minutes.

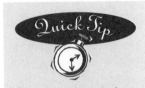

To remove kernels from a corn cob, set the corn cob upright on a cutting board and slice off 2 to 3 rows of kernels with a sharp knife.

Samosas

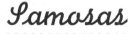

3 cups frozen chopped hash
  brown potatoes
¾ cup frozen peas
1 onion, chopped
⅓ cup water
1 teaspoon minced fresh
  garlic

½ teaspoon minced fresh
  gingerroot
1½ teaspoons curry powder
½ teaspoon ground coriander
1 teaspoon soy sauce
15 sheets Amber Farms Spinach
  Pasta Wraps

*Servings: makes 15
Preparation Time:
15 minutes
Cooking Time:
38 minutes*

Preheat the oven to 350 degrees.

Place the potatoes in a saucepan with water to cover. Cover, bring to a boil, and cook over medium heat for 5 minutes. Add the peas and cook for 2 minutes longer. Remove from heat and drain.

Meanwhile, place the onion, water, garlic, and gingerroot in another pan. Cook, stirring occasionally, for 5 minutes. Add the curry powder, coriander and soy sauce. Cook for 1 minute. Remove from heat.

Combine the potato mixture with the onion mixture and mix well.

Take one sheet of the pasta wraps and place it so that one of the points faces you. Place 1 heaping tablespoon of the mixture in the center of the wrap. Fold up the bottom, then fold in the sides. Moisten the top triangle with water, then fold over the top point to seal. Place seam side down on a nonstick or parchment paper–covered baking sheet. Bake for 15 minutes, turn over, and bake for another 10 minutes.

Recipe Hint: *You can prepare these samosas ahead of time and bake later. They may even be frozen before baking, but be sure to thaw completely before baking. Pack them in lunches or take on a picnic. Serve hot or cold with one of the tofu dip recipes in this book, such as Curry Tofu Dip (page 258) or Creamy Cilantro-Garlic Dressing (page 49). We like them with Cilantro Pesto (page 215). Amber Farms Spinach Pasta Wraps are made by JSL Foods, Inc., in Los Angeles, California. They are similar to egg roll wrappers and are made from flour, water, and spinach. They are sold in packages of 20 and are about 5 inches square.*

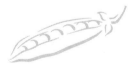

Oriental Wraps

Servings: makes 11
Preparation Time:
15 minutes
Cooking Time:
35 minutes

⅓ cup water
1 onion, chopped
1 teaspoon minced fresh
    garlic
1 teaspoon minced fresh
    gingerroot
1 cup sliced fresh mushrooms
½ cup finely chopped celery
½ cup finely chopped green or
    red bell pepper

¼ cup sliced water chestnuts, cut
    into thin strips
2 green onions, thinly sliced
dash of sesame oil (optional)
2 tablespoons soy sauce
1 tablespoon mirin
1 tablespoon cornstarch mixed
    with 2 tablespoons cold water
11 sheets Amber Farms Spinach
    Pasta Wraps

Preheat the oven to 350 degrees.

Place the water, onion, garlic, and gingerroot in a medium non-stick frying pan. Cook, stirring occasionally, for 5 minutes. Add the mushrooms, celery, bell pepper, water chestnuts, green onions, and sesame oil, if using. Cook, stirring frequently, for 5 minutes. Stir in the soy sauce and mirin. Add the cornstarch mixture while stirring; cook and stir until thickened and well mixed.

Take one sheet of the pasta wraps and place it so that one of the points faces you. Place 1 heaping tablespoon of the mixture in the center of the wrap. Fold up the bottom, then fold in the sides. Moisten the top triangle with water, then fold over the top point to seal. Place seam side down on a nonstick or parchment paper–covered baking sheet. Bake for 15 minutes, turn over, and bake for another 10 minutes.

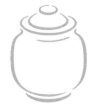

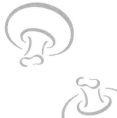

Recipe Hint: Serve hot or cold with Sweet and Sour Dipping Sauce (page 218) or Oriental Dipping Sauce (page 218). You can prepare them ahead of time and bake later. Our daughter used to like to take them to school for lunch.

Empanadas

⅓ cup water
1 onion, chopped
½ cup chopped green bell pepper
½ teaspoon minced fresh garlic
2 teaspoons chili powder
½ teaspoon ground cumin

1 15-ounce can nonfat refried
  beans
dash or two of Tabasco sauce
14 sheets Amber Farms Spinach
  Pasta Wraps

Servings: makes 14
Preparation Time:
  15 minutes
Cooking Time:
  30 minutes

Preheat the oven to 350 degrees.

Place the water, onion, bell pepper, and garlic in a medium non-stick frying pan. Cook, stirring occasionally, for 7 minutes. Add the chili powder and cumin and cook for another minute. Add the beans and Tabasco sauce. Mix well and heat through, about 2 minutes.

Take one sheet of the pasta wraps and place it so that one of the points faces you. Place 1 heaping tablespoon of the mixture in the center of the wrap. Fold up the bottom, then fold in the sides. Moisten the top triangle with water, then fold over the top point to seal. Place seam side down on a nonstick or parchment paper-covered baking sheet. Bake for 10 minutes, turn over, and bake for another 10 minutes.

Recipe Hint: *You can prepare these empanadas ahead and bake later. Serve plain, hot or cold, or dip in salsa, if desired.*

Spring Rolls

Servings: 12
Preparation Time:
15 minutes
Chilling Time:
1 hour

1 cup shredded cabbage
½ cup finely chopped firm tofu
¼ cup finely chopped water
 chestnuts
¼ cup mung bean sprouts

⅛ cup finely chopped green
 onions
3½ tablespoons plum sauce
dash of sesame oil (optional)
3 nonfat flour tortillas

Combine the cabbage, tofu, water chestnuts, mung bean sprouts, green onions, 2½ tablespoons of the plum sauce, and the sesame oil, if using, in a bowl. Mix gently to coat. Spread the remaining 1 tablespoon plum sauce thinly over the tortillas, leaving a small edge on each one. Spread the cabbage mixture evenly over the plum sauce on each tortilla. Roll up tightly. Place each roll on a square of parchment paper and roll tightly again. Twist the ends of the parchment paper to seal well. Refrigerate at least 1 hour before serving.

When ready to serve, unwrap, cut off a small amount of the ends, and then cut each roll into 4 pieces.

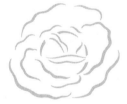

Recipe Hint: *These taste better if made 1 day ahead to allow the tofu to pick up more flavor. This recipe is easily doubled.*

ETHNIC SEASONINGS

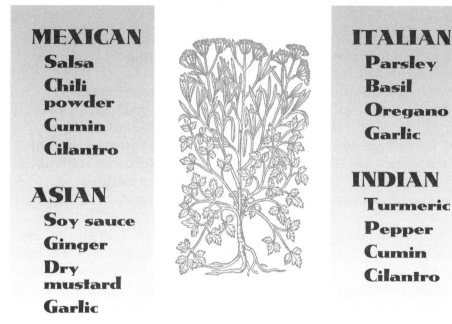

MEXICAN
Salsa
Chili
powder
Cumin
Cilantro

ASIAN
Soy sauce
Ginger
Dry
mustard
Garlic

ITALIAN
Parsley
Basil
Oregano
Garlic

INDIAN
Turmeric
Pepper
Cumin
Cilantro

*S*easoning makes a dish interesting and enjoyable. You should pick familiar spices to use in your cooking. The same rice, bean, or noodle dish can be made to taste Mexican, Italian, Asian, or Indian by choosing various combinations of spices.

People love salt and sugar for a very good reason: The tip of our tongue has taste buds that are pleased by these two substances. We are designed as seekers of sweet-tasting carbohydrates. Rice, corn, potatoes, fruits, and maybe a little honey provided sweetness in the past. Now manufacturers dump 150 pounds of sugar per person into our yearly food supply to satisfy our "sweet tooth." Salt-seeking taste buds are looking for once-rare essential minerals. Today every dining table has a salt shaker on it that provides an excess of minerals in the form of sodium chloride.

In order to get the most pleasure from salt and sugar, with the least risk to your health, you should sprinkle the flavoring on the surface of the food, where your tongue can easily contact it, just before eating. When salt and sugar are added during cooking, most of the flavor is lost, but they have the same effect on your body whether or not you taste them.

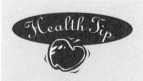

Garlic and red peppers are enjoyable flavorings that lower cholesterol and benefit the cardiovascular system by thinning the blood, preventing the blood clots that produce heart attacks.

Moo-Shu Wraps

Servings: 8
Preparation Time:
15 minutes
Cooking Time:
15 minutes

½ cup water
2 cups shredded napa cabbage or
   regular cabbage
1 cup sliced fresh mushrooms
1 red bell pepper, cut into thin
   strips
1 cup mung bean sprouts
4 green onions, cut into short
   thin strips
½ cup shredded carrots

1 teaspoon minced fresh garlic
2 teaspoons minced fresh
   gingerroot
3 tablespoons soy sauce
1 10.5-ounce package lite firm
   tofu, cut into strips
1 tablespoon cornstarch mixed
   with 2 tablespoons cold water
8 fat-free flour tortillas
⅓ cup plum sauce

Place the water in a large nonstick frying pan. Add all the vegetables, the garlic, and ginger. Cook, stirring frequently, for 5 minutes. Add the soy sauce and tofu, cook, and stir for 5 more minutes. Stir in the cornstarch mixture. Cook and stir until thickened. Place a line of the vegetable mixture down the center of each tortilla. Spoon a little plum sauce over the vegetables. Roll up and eat.

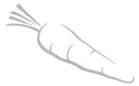

Recipe Hint: *Buy presliced mushrooms, shredded carrots, and shredded cabbage to save time, or shred carrots, zucchini, celery, and cucumbers with the large holes of a grater.*

Pizza

½ cup fat-free bottled Italian-
  style sauce
1 large Kabuli Pizza Crust

assorted toppings: chopped
  onions, chopped green
  peppers, sliced mushrooms,
  chopped pineapple, chopped
  zucchini, chopped broccoli,
  chopped spinach, artichoke
  hearts

Servings: 8
Preparation Time:
5 to 10 minutes
Cooking Time:
10 to 12 minutes

Preheat the oven to 450 degrees.

Spread the sauce evenly over the pizza crust. Add the toppings of
your choice. Place on a baking tray and bake for 10 to 11 minutes,
until the crust is golden.

Recipe Hint: *Kabuli Pizza Crust is made by Dallas Gourmet Bakery and can be found in natural food stores. It contains flour, yeast, and salt. There are many fat-free Italian sauces available in natural foods stores and supermarkets. Use a marinara, spaghetti, or pizza sauce for a traditional taste. Experiment with other sauces, such as enchilada, curry, or Szechwan.*

Mexican Pizza

Servings: 8
Preparation Time:
10 minutes
Cooking Time:
12 minutes

1¼ cups nonfat refried beans
1 large Kabuli Pizza Crust
1 cup salsa
¼ cup chopped onion
¼ cup chopped tomatoes

⅛ cup sliced black olives
   (optional)
1 tablespoon chopped canned
   green chilies
1 cup shredded lettuce

Preheat the oven to 450 degrees.

Spread the beans over the crust. Spread ⅓ cup of the salsa over the beans. Layer the onion, tomatoes, olives, and chilies over the beans and salsa. Bake for 12 minutes, until the crust is golden.

Remove the pizza from the oven. Layer with the lettuce and top with the remaining salsa.

Black Bean Pizza

Servings: 8
Preparation Time:
10 minutes
Cooking Time:
10 to 12 minutes

¾ cup tomato sauce
½ teaspoon ground cumin
½ teaspoon garlic powder
½ teaspoon thyme
1 large Kabuli Pizza Crust

1 15-ounce can black beans,
   drained and rinsed
1 cup frozen corn kernels, thawed
1 onion, chopped
½ cup salsa

Preheat the oven to 450 degrees.

Combine the tomato sauce, cumin, garlic powder, and thyme. Spread over the pizza crust. Combine the black beans, corn, onion, and salsa. Spoon evenly over the pizza crust on top of the tomato sauce. Bake for 10 to 12 minutes, until the crust is golden.

Recipe Hint: For those of you who like a little "heat," add a few chopped or sliced jalapeños to the bean mixture. Kabuli Pizza Crust is made by Dallas Gourmet Bakery.

Peppered Black Pizza

1 15-ounce can black beans,
   drained and rinsed
1 teaspoon minced fresh garlic
⅛ cup water
1 tomato, chopped
2 dashes of Tabasco sauce
½ cup canned roasted peppers,
   chopped

¼ cup sliced green olives
¼ cup sliced ripe black olives
½ teaspoon crushed red
   pepper
1 large Kabuli Pizza Crust
1 small avocado, sliced
   (optional)

Servings: 8
Preparation Time:
   15 minutes
Cooking Time:
   12 minutes

Preheat the oven to 450 degrees.

Place the black beans and garlic in a food processor and process briefly. Add the water while processing and process until smooth. Transfer to a small bowl. Add the tomato and Tabasco sauce. Mix and set aside.

Combine the roasted peppers, olives, and crushed red pepper. Drain excess liquid. Spread the bean mixture over the crust. Spoon the olive mixture over the bean spread. Arrange a few slices of avocado over the pizza, if desired. Bake for 12 minutes, until the crust is golden.

Recipe Hint: This is a very interesting variation on a bean pizza, mainly because of the pepper and olive mixture. To jazz this up even more, add some chopped cilantro to the olive mixture, between ⅛ to ¼ cup. You can also add some shredded soy cheese before baking.

PRESSURE COOKERS

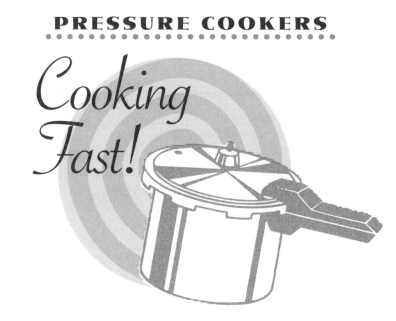

Cooking Fast!

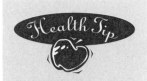
One convenient, low-cost way to cook healthy foods quickly is to use a pressure cooker. The jiggle-top cookers release steam throughout the cooking process, creating noise and releasing odor and steam into the kitchen. The newer cookers use a valve that releases steam only when the pressure is greater than needed for cooking (and the heat should then be turned down); they require little liquid and are silent. Older cookers had to be cooled under water before opening; however, the newer ones don't. Newer models are much more expensive.

In general, foods cook in one third to one half the time required by conventional cooking. Err on the side of undercooking, and use 20 percent less liquid for soups and stews. The longer the food ordinarily has to cook the greater the time savings; thus pressure cookers are great for beans, peas, lentils, and some grains. Times to cook ingredients are listed in the instruction booklet that comes with your cooker. Correct timing is essential, because a few extra minutes can ruin a recipe. The best recipes for a pressure cooker are ones that are cooked on the stovetop and those that combine most of the ingredients at the beginning. Use about 50 percent more spices and herbs than the recipe calls for because this intense cooking diminishes their flavors.

White Bean Pizza

1 15-ounce can white beans, drained and rinsed
1 teaspoon lemon juice
⅛ teaspoon garlic powder
several twists of freshly ground black pepper
1 large Kabuli Pizza Crust
1 8-ounce can pineapple chunks, drained

1 tomato, chopped
1 cup coarsely chopped fresh spinach
½ cup thinly sliced zucchini
1 to 2 teaspoons minced fresh garlic

Servings: 8
Preparation Time:
15 minutes
Cooking Time:
12 minutes

Preheat the oven to 450 degrees.

Place the beans, lemon juice, garlic powder, and pepper in a food processor and process until smooth. Spread over the pizza crust. Arrange the pineapple, tomato, spinach, zucchini, and garlic over the bean spread. Bake for 12 minutes, until the crust is golden.

Recipe Hint: *To "jazz up" the bean spread, add ½ to 1 teaspoon of Tabasco sauce while processing.*

Vegetable Pizzas

Servings: 8
Preparation Time:
15 minutes
Cooking Time:
12 to 14 minutes

4 whole wheat pita breads
½ cup water
1 onion, sliced and separated
  into rings
1 green bell pepper, chopped
2½ cups chopped fresh tomatoes
½ teaspoon minced fresh garlic
½ teaspoon basil

½ teaspoon oregano
¼ teaspoon thyme
¼ teaspoon marjoram
1 teaspoon sugar
2 tablespoons cornstarch
½ cup grated soy cheese
  (optional)

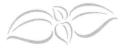

Preheat the oven to 375 degrees.

Cut each pita bread along the sides and split into 2 circles. Place the inside up and bake on a nonstick baking sheet for 8 minutes.

Meanwhile, place ¼ cup of the water in a saucepan with the onion and bell pepper. Cook, stirring occasionally, for 2 minutes. Add the tomatoes, garlic, and all the seasonings. Bring to a boil, reduce heat, cover, and simmer for 6 minutes. Combine the cornstarch with the remaining ¼ cup water. Stir into the vegetable mixture and cook and stir until the mixture boils and thickens. Remove from heat.

Spread the vegetable mixture over the pita halves. Sprinkle with cheese, if desired. Bake for another 3 to 4 minutes.

Recipe Hint: You can make these pizzas with fat-free flour tortillas. The flour tortillas will bake in 3 to 4 minutes.

Polenta with Mushrooms

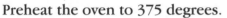

1 24-ounce package precooked
  polenta
⅓ cup water
2 tablespoons sherry
1 tablespoon soy sauce
½ pound fresh shiitake
  mushrooms, sliced
½ pound fresh cremini
  mushrooms, sliced
¼ pound fresh oyster
  mushrooms, sliced

1 small onion, chopped
1 teaspoon minced fresh
  garlic
1 tablespoon thinly sliced fresh
  basil
1 tablespoon chopped fresh
  parsley
several twists of freshly ground
  black pepper

Servings: 4
Preparation Time:
15 minutes
Cooking Time:
15 minutes

Preheat the oven to 375 degrees.

Slice the polenta into ½-inch-thick slices. Place on a nonstick baking sheet and bake for 15 minutes.

Meanwhile, place all the remaining ingredients in a nonstick frying pan and cook, stirring occasionally, for 10 minutes.

Serve the mushrooms over the baked polenta.

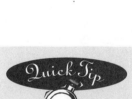

Quick Tip

Found on supermarket shelves, ready-made polenta rolls are a traditional Italian corn-based alternative to pasta, bread, or rice. Microwave for 60 to 90 seconds, brown on a nonstick griddle for 5 to 10 minutes, or bake in an oven for 15 minutes. Serve plain or top warm polenta with sauces and salsas. Polenta is delicious with many different sauces.

Polenta with Italian Bean Sauce

Servings: 4
Preparation Time:
10 minutes
Cooking Time:
20 minutes

1 24-ounce package precooked polenta
⅓ cup water
1 onion, chopped
1 green bell pepper, chopped
½ teaspoon minced fresh garlic
1 15-ounce can garbanzo beans, drained and rinsed

1 15-ounce can white beans, drained and rinsed
1 14.5-ounce can Italian-style stewed tomatoes
1½ cups frozen cut green beans

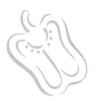

Preheat the oven to 375 degrees.

Slice the polenta into ½-inch-thick slices. Place on a nonstick baking sheet and bake for 15 minutes.

Meanwhile, place the water, onion, bell pepper, and garlic in a saucepan. Cook, stirring occasionally, for 5 minutes. Add the garbanzo beans, white beans, and tomatoes. Cook for another 10 minutes. Add the green beans and cook an additional 5 minutes, stirring occasionally.

Serve over the polenta.

Recipe Hint: Found on supermarket shelves, ready-made polenta rolls are a traditional Italian corn-based alternative to pasta, bread, or rice. Microwave for 60 to 90 seconds, brown on a nonstick griddle for 5 to 10 minutes, or bake in an oven for 15 minutes. Serve plain or top warm polenta with sauces and salsas. This sauce is also delicious over pasta.

Seitan Curry

1 small onion, chopped
½ cup water
2½ teaspoons minced fresh
   gingerroot
⅓ cup unbleached flour

4 cups soy or rice milk
2 to 3 teaspoons curry powder
1½ tablespoons lemon juice
8 ounces chopped seitan, turkey-
   or chicken-style

Servings: 4 to 6
Preparation Time:
15 minutes
Cooking Time:
30 minutes

Put the onion and water in a large saucepan. Cook and stir until the onion softens slightly, add ginger, and cook for 2 minutes. Turn off heat. Stir in the flour. Gradually add 1 cup of the milk while stirring. Turn heat on low and cook very gently for 2 minutes, stirring constantly. Add the remaining 3 cups milk and the other ingredients. Cook, uncovered, over very low heat for 25 minutes, stirring occasionally. The mixture will thicken as it slowly cooks. Serve over rice with assorted condiments (chopped green onions, raisins, drained chopped pineapple, mandarin orange segments) to spoon over the top, if desired.

Recipe Hint: *Harmony Farms Fat-Free Rice Drink works well in this recipe.*

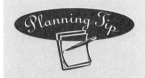

Many cookbooks tell you to gather all the ingredients before you start cooking. We suggest you get started with a job like sautéing onions and then gather other ingredients and do other tasks.

MICROWAVE COOKING

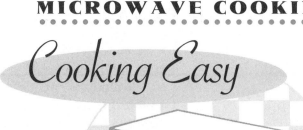

Cooking Easy

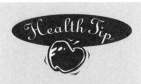

Raw foods have some nutritional advantages. Because they're less digestible they cause greater weight loss and lower blood sugar levels. However, cooking enhances the flavor of most foods, and many foods like rice and dried beans must be cooked to be soft enough to eat.

The advantages of microwave cooking are cost and time savings. We use the microwave in our home mostly for rewarming leftovers, baking one or two potatoes, reheating vegetarian burgers, cooking frozen vegetables, boiling water for instant cup soups, and refreshing bread products. Microwave cooking leaves dishes moist.

You can convert saucy dishes and stews in this book to cook in the microwave. Begin by cooking the dish on high for one quarter as long as stated in the recipe. Since little evaporation occurs, reduce the amount of liquid called for in the recipe by one quarter. Cover all foods cooked in the microwave to hold in the steam and help cook faster without drying out. For even cooking, stir the food occasionally and rotate the dish several times. Microwaved food continues to cook after it is removed from the oven. Microwave cooking does not damage the food any more than conventional cooking. In fact, nutrient content is often higher in microwaved foods. However, you should be sure that your microwave does not leak radiation that might affect your health. Buy an inexpensive radiation leakage detector and check the door seal for leakage.

Baked Tofu Loaf

1 pound tofu, mashed
1½ cups quick-cooking oatmeal
¼ cup ketchup
¼ cup parsley flakes

2 tablespoons onion flakes
½ teaspoon garlic powder
several twists of freshly ground
    black pepper

Preheat the oven to 350 degrees.

Combine all ingredients in a bowl and mix well. Pack into a non-stick 9 × 5-inch loaf pan. Bake for 30 minutes. Let cool for 5 minutes before removing from the pan.

Serve with mashed potatoes and gravy.

Servings: 8
Preparation Time:
10 minutes
Cooking Time:
30 minutes

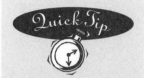

In a microwave, casseroles and baked dishes cook in one-fourth the time they take in a conventional oven. Time, energy, costs, and nutrients are saved. Be sure that the door's seal is tight with a micro-wave-leakage detector to avoid exposure to the microwaves.

Recipe Hint: *You can make this loaf ahead of time and refrigerate until ready to bake.*

Microwaved Ratatouille

1 onion, sliced and separated
    into rings
1 green bell pepper, coarsely
    chopped
2 zucchini, thinly sliced

1 eggplant, cut into cubes
½ teaspoon minced fresh garlic
2 tomatoes, coarsely chopped
1 teaspoon dried basil leaves
1 teaspoon dried oregano leaves

¼ teaspoon dried thyme
several twists of freshly ground black pepper

Combine all ingredients in a microwave-safe dish. Cover. Micro-wave on high for 10 minutes, stirring every 3 minutes. Serve hot over baked potatoes, grains, or pasta, or serve cold as a salad.

Servings: 6
Preparation Time:
15 minutes
Cooking Time:
10 minutes

Thai Tofu with Cashews

Servings: 2
Preparation Time:
10 minutes
Cooking Time:
10 minutes

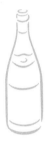

5 tablespoons soy sauce

5 tablespoons dry sherry

5 tablespoons water

1½ teaspoons minced fresh garlic

1 teaspoon minced fresh
gingerroot

1 teaspoon crushed red pepper

2 tablespoons cornstarch

1 bunch green onions, chopped

1 10.5-ounce package firm lite
silken tofu, cubed

⅓ cup cashew pieces

Combine the soy sauce, sherry, water, garlic, ginger, and red pepper in a small bowl. Mix well. Pour about two-thirds of the liquid into a nonstick frying pan; reserve the rest. Add the cornstarch to the reserved liquid and set aside.

Add the green onions, tofu, and cashews to the frying pan. Cook, stirring frequently, until the mixture is bubbling, about 8 minutes. Stir in the cornstarch mixture and continue to cook and stir until thickened, about 2 minutes.

Serve over rice or pasta.

Recipe Hint: *Try adding ½ cup diced, lightly cooked zucchini to the mixture after it has thickened.*

Baked Seasoned Tofu

1 10.5-ounce package lite extra-firm silken tofu, frozen and thawed (see hint)
2 tablespoons soy sauce
1 teaspoon poultry seasoning
1 teaspoon nutritional yeast powder
1 teaspoon lime juice
½ teaspoon minced fresh garlic
¼ teaspoon minced fresh gingerroot

Servings: 6
Preparation Time: 5 minutes (need thawed frozen tofu)
Marinating Time: 30 minutes
Baking Time: 40 minutes

Cut the tofu into 6 slices lengthwise. Combine the remaining ingredients in a rectangular baking dish. Marinate the tofu in the sauce for 30 minutes, turning several times.

Preheat the oven to 350 degrees.

Bake for 40 minutes, turning once halfway through the baking time. Add to sandwiches or eat plain.

Recipe Hint: *Freezing changes tofu from a soft cheesy consistency to a chewy meatlike texture. To freeze tofu, place the unopened package in the freezer for at least 1 day. To thaw, remove from the freezer and let thaw at room temperature for 6 hours. To quick thaw, place the package in a bowl and cover with boiling water. Remove the tofu from the package, squeeze out excess water, and slice.*

Tofu Jambalaya

Servings: 4
Preparation Time:
15 minutes
Cooking Time:
15 minutes

1 cup uncooked orzo
⅓ cup water
1 onion, chopped
1 green bell pepper, chopped
2 stalks celery, chopped
1 teaspoon minced fresh garlic
1 14.5-ounce can chopped
  tomatoes
2 bay leaves
½ teaspoon thyme

¼ teaspoon dry mustard
several twists of freshly ground
  black pepper
several dashes of Tabasco
  sauce
1 6.5-ounce package Smoked
  Tofu, diced
1 15-ounce can kidney beans,
  drained and rinsed
2 green onions, chopped

Put a large pot of water on to boil. Drop the orzo into boiling water and cook according to the package directions.

Meanwhile, place the water, onion, bell pepper, celery, and garlic in a saucepan. Cook, stirring occasionally, for 5 minutes. Add the tomatoes, bay leaves, thyme, mustard, pepper, and Tabasco sauce. Bring to a boil, reduce heat, and simmer, uncovered, for 10 minutes. Remove the bay leaves. Add the tofu, beans, and cooked orzo. Heat through and serve with the green onions sprinkled over the top.

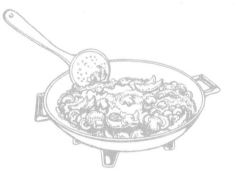

Tofu Burgers

2 10.5-ounce packages lite firm
   silken tofu
2½ cups quick-cooking oatmeal
1½ tablespoons soy sauce
1½ tablespoons Worcestershire
   sauce

1½ tablespoons prepared
   mustard
1½ tablespoons fat-free garlic
   sauce, barbecue sauce, or other
   spicy sauce

Servings: 9
Preparation Time:
15 minutes
Cooking Time:
30 minutes

Preheat the oven to 350 degrees.

Place the tofu in a large bowl and mash well. Stir in the oatmeal and the seasonings. Mix well. Form into patties and place on a non-stick baking tray. Bake for 20 minutes, turn over, and bake for an additional 10 minutes.

Serve on whole wheat buns with all the trimmings.

Recipe Hint: These are the burgers John and son Craig eat when they play paintball. Mary puts the burger inside a whole wheat bun, packs it in a plastic bag, and sends condiments along for them to add at lunchtime. It's a great take-along lunch. The burgers are easy to make ahead of time and they store well in the refrigerator or freezer. After they are baked, they may be grilled, either plain or with some teriyaki sauce brushed on both sides.

Spinach Buns

Servings: 6
Preparation Time:
15 minutes
Cooking Time:
2 minutes

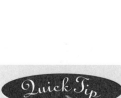

1 15-ounce can garbanzo beans, drained and rinsed
¼ cup lemon juice
2 tablespoons water
1 tablespoon capers
1 tablespoon balsamic vinegar
½ teaspoon minced fresh garlic
1 6-ounce bag washed baby spinach
several twists of freshly ground black pepper
6 whole wheat buns

Place the garbanzo beans, lemon juice, water, and capers in a food processor and process until smooth.

Place the vinegar in a medium saucepan. Add the garlic. Stir for 1 minute. Add the spinach and stir for another minute. Season with the pepper.

Split the buns in half. Spread the garbanzo mixture evenly over the top and bottom of the buns. Place the spinach mixture in between, close up, and eat.

Quick Tip

Steaming vegetables in one of those collapsible baskets is often frustrating: The basket often folds at a critical moment. Instead, use a stainless steel pot with an insert with holes to steam all your vegetables. Remove the insert and pour the vegetables into a bowl.

SLOW COOKERS

Convenience

The art of slow cooking has almost been lost. It's time to get out your Crock-Pot to cut down your workload. In the morning, before you get your day going, you can make dinner, or at night, before you go to bed, you can start breakfast. The whole house will take on the delicious aromas of your meals. Slow cooking blends flavors and keeps the kitchen cool in warm weather. It's almost impossible to overcook and foods don't stick to the bottom. Vegetables, grains, and beans are ideal for slow cookers.

Use whole leaf herbs and increase the amount of herbs and spices the recipe calls for because some of their flavor is lost by prolonged cooking. Cook with the lid on to prevent moisture loss and hold heat. Resist looking inside because of substantial heat loss. To adapt a favorite recipe, estimate three to four hours on low setting, or two to two and a half on high for each hour of conventional cooking. One pound of beans takes eight and a half to ten hours on low heat; split peas and lentils take about three and a half hours on low heat.

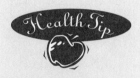

Cooking breaks down complex carbohydrates into simpler sugars that have a sweet, pleasurable taste. Cooking also destroys toxic substances, such as trypsin inhibitors in raw soybeans.

Spicy White Bean Pitas

Servings: 6 to 8
Preparation Time:
10 minutes
Cooking Time:
15 minutes

1 onion, chopped
⅓ cup water
2 15-ounce cans white beans,
  drained and rinsed
2 10-ounce cans diced tomatoes
  and chilies

1 cup frozen corn kernels
⅓ cup tomato paste
2 teaspoons chili powder
6 to 8 pita breads
1 bunch chopped green onions
1 cup alfalfa sprouts

Cook the onion in the water for 5 minutes, stirring occasionally. Add the beans, tomatoes, corn, tomato paste, and chili powder. Cook, uncovered, over medium heat for 10 minutes, stirring occasionally. Serve in pita breads, topped with the green onions and sprouts.

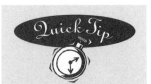

To chop onions quickly, cut both ends off, then cut in half lengthwise. Place one half cut side down, turn and make crosswise slices, then turn and cut lengthwise to chop into cubes.

Grilled Portobello Mushrooms

4 large portobello mushrooms
¼ cup balsamic vinegar *or*
  soy sauce

1 teaspoon minced fresh garlic
several twists of freshly ground
  black pepper

Servings: 4
Preparation Time:
5 minutes
Cooking Time:
10 minutes

Clean the mushrooms well and leave whole or slice thickly crosswise. Combine remaining ingredients in a small bowl. Brush mushrooms with this mixture on both sides and grill over medium coals for about 5 minutes on each side. Brush with more of the mixture while grilling. Serve at once.

Recipe Hint: *Whole portobello mushrooms make delicious burgers. Serve them on a whole wheat bun with lettuce, tomatoes, onions, ketchup, and mustard. They have a wonderful meaty taste and texture. For variety, we sometimes brush teriyaki sauce over the mushrooms before grilling. These mushrooms are a staple in our home during the summer months, and they have become a favorite among friends and relatives too.*

Grilled Red Potatoes

6 medium red potatoes, scrubbed

1 to 2 teaspoons Cajun seasoning mix

Servings: 4
Preparation Time: 3 minutes
Cooking Time: 20 minutes

Place the potatoes on a paper towel in a microwave oven. Cook for 5 minutes on one side, turn over and cook for another 5 minutes. The potatoes should be tender, but not too soft. Remove and place in a bowl of cold water. Drain and pat dry. Cut the potatoes in half lengthwise and carefully thread onto skewers. Sprinkle the cut side with seasoning mix. Place on a grill over medium coals and grill for 5 minutes on each side, until tender and brown.

Recipe Hint: Other seasoning blends may also be used, such as chili powder, Italian, or another favorite blend. There are many varieties sold in supermarkets. Vary the amount of potatoes used for more or less servings. We eat these with ketchup or various barbecue sauces through the summer months whenever we use our grill. If you do not have skewers, the potatoes may be placed directly on the grill and turned with a spatula or tongs.

Southwest Red Potatoes

Servings: 4
Preparation Time:
10 minutes
Cooking Time:
15 minutes

2 1-pound bags frozen whole red
  potatoes
¼ cup chopped green onions
¼ cup oil-free salad dressing

¾ teaspoon chili powder
¾ teaspoon ground cumin
⅛ teaspoon red pepper flakes

Boil the potatoes in water to cover for 10 minutes. Drain. Cut into chunks. Place the remaining ingredients in a nonstick frying pan. Add the potatoes and cook until coated with spices, about 5 minutes.

Sweet Potatoes and Apples

Servings: 4
Preparation Time:
10 minutes
Cooking Time:
40 minutes

1 large baking apple, peeled and
  sliced
2 medium sweet potatoes, peeled
  and thinly sliced

½ cup applesauce
½ cup water
½ teaspoon cinnamon

Preheat the oven to 400 degrees.
Layer the apple and sweet potatoes in a square baking dish. Combine the applesauce and water and pour over the layered ingredients. Sprinkle with the cinnamon. Cover and bake at 400 degrees for 40 minutes. Serve hot or cold.

Quick Tip

In four to five minutes you can cook white or sweet potatoes in a microwave on high. With a fork, poke many holes through the skin before cooking or they will explode.

Rainbow Skillet Medley

5 cups frozen chopped hash
  brown potatoes
5 cups water
2 cups chopped broccoli
½ cup vegetable broth
½ teaspoon minced fresh garlic
1 bunch green onions, chopped
1 red bell pepper, chopped

1 green bell pepper, chopped
1 cup frozen corn kernels
1 teaspoon basil
1 teaspoon oregano
½ teaspoon dill weed
several twists of freshly ground
  black pepper
dash or two of Tabasco sauce

Servings: 4
Preparation Time:
15 minutes
Cooking Time:
20 minutes

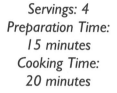

Place the potatoes and water in a medium pot. Bring to a boil. Add the broccoli, cover, and cook for 5 minutes. Drain.

Place the vegetable broth and garlic in a large nonstick frying pan. Heat to boiling, then add the potatoes, broccoli, and the remaining ingredients. Cook, stirring frequently, for 10 minutes.

Recipe Hint: *Serve hot as a complete meal. Roll up in a tortilla or stuff into pita bread. Sprinkle with some salsa or Tabasco sauce for a spicy flavor.*

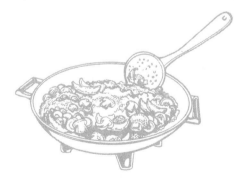

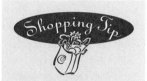

Plan your menus for the week. Make a shopping list. Avoid last-minute decisions, impulse buying, and repeat trips to the store for forgotten items.

POTATOES—
FAST & EASY

Potatoes

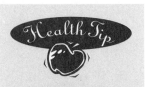

Health Tip

Potatoes can be complete nutrition. After six months of a diet where all the nutrients came from potatoes, a man and woman were declared in excellent health—they did, however, lose lots of weight.

The fastest way to have cooked potatoes is to use precooked frozen potatoes. They are found in the frozen food section of your grocery in boxes or bags (see the canned and packaged products list on page 286). You can buy them unpeeled, peeled, chopped, or shredded. Our favorite frozen potatoes are loose shredded and shredded compacted into rectangles that we cook in a nonstick pan as hash browns. Top with barbecue sauce, tomato relish, or steak sauce to give them a great taste (see the canned and packaged products list on page 286). Adding frozen chopped potatoes to soups and stews is an easy way to thicken them. Sliced and whole white potatoes are also sold in cans, as are sweet potatoes, but they are packed in a sugar syrup.

Raw potatoes can be microwaved in ten minutes, baked in an hour, and boiled in twenty minutes depending on their size. There are many varieties of potatoes that serve well as the foundation of your starch-based meal plan.

Sauces

Cilantro Pesto

4 cups cilantro leaves
¼ cup cashews
1 tablespoon lemon juice

1 teaspoon soy sauce
½ tablespoon water

Place all ingredients, except the water, in a food processor. Process until smooth, adding the water a little at a time, if necessary.

> *Recipe Hint:* *Use 1 tablespoon of pesto at a time to add flavor to salad dressings, pasta, and grains. This pesto has a very strong flavor and probably will appeal only to cilantro lovers. We use this as a spread for crackers and fat-free crumpets.*

*Servings: makes
1 cup
Preparation Time:
5 minutes*

Basil Pesto

4 cups basil leaves
2 teaspoons minced fresh garlic
¼ cup pine nuts

1 teaspoon soy sauce
1 tablespoon water

Place all ingredients, except the water, in a food processor. Process until smooth, adding the water a little at a time.

> *Recipe Hint:* *Use 1 tablespoon of pesto at a time to add flavor to salad dressings. Mix it into grain salads or stir into hot pasta. Pesto is usually made with olive oil and cheese, so this is a much healthier alternative.*

*Servings: makes
1 ½ cups
Preparation Time:
5 minutes*

GLOBAL DIFFERENCES

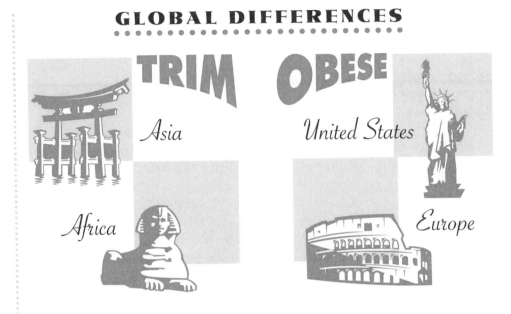

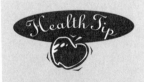

Chinese consume more calories than Americans, yet they are always trim. Their calories mostly come from complex carbohydrates, ours mostly from fat and sugar. Food is not your enemy ... the more you eat of the right foods the thinner and healthier you will become.

A look around the world provides you with incontrovertible evidence of the cause of common diseases. Obesity is common in wealthy countries; Americans and Western Europeans suffer from heart disease, hypertension, diabetes, rheumatoid arthritis and multiple sclerosis, and breast, prostate, and colon cancers. In the underdeveloped countries of Africa and Asia, people are trim and avoid these chronic diseases. They live on diets centered around starches—rice, corn, potatoes, beans—with fruits and vegetables. Meat and dairy products are a very small part of their diet, if at all.

But things are changing. To find a "better life" millions of people are migrating to the wealthy nations in North America and Europe. After they move, they usually change their diets, becoming fatter and sicker. We are now exporting our fast food and "all you can eat" styles of living to the rest of the world, and as a result their health is declining.

Science has conquered most of the diseases common to people of underdeveloped countries by advances in sanitation, immunization, and medicine. You and your family can enjoy the benefits of modern living, personal wealth, and technology without suffering the health problems they can bring by eating the diet humans were designed to thrive on—a starch-based diet with vegetables and fruits.

Tofu Pesto

1 cup fresh basil leaves
¼ cup raw cashews
3 to 4 teaspoons minced fresh
   garlic

1 10.5-ounce package lite silken
   tofu
1 to 2 tablespoons soy parmesan
   cheese (optional)

Servings: makes
2 cups
Preparation Time:
10 minutes

    Place the basil, cashews, and garlic in a food processor. Process until smooth. Add the tofu and cheese, if desired, and process until smooth and creamy.

> **Recipe Hint:** *This is good mixed with pasta, used as a pizza sauce, spread on crackers or bread, or used as a salad dressing. Cut down on the fat by making it without the cashews.*

Oriental Dipping Sauce

Servings: makes
½ cup
Preparation Time:
2 minutes

¼ to ½ teaspoon wasabi   ½ cup soy sauce

Place the wasabi in the bottom of a bowl. (Wasabi can be quite hot, so use the lesser amount if you are unfamiliar with it.) Add a small amount of the soy sauce and mix until the wasabi and soy sauce are very smooth, adding a little more soy sauce if necessary. Add the remaining soy sauce and mix until well blended.

> ***Recipe Hint:*** *Wasabi is a green Japanese horseradish paste found in Asian markets and sometimes supermarkets. It is traditionally mixed with soy sauce to make a seasoning for sushi. Wasabi can be very hot, so use sparingly.*

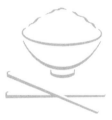

Sweet and Sour Dipping Sauce

Servings: makes
1 cup
Preparation Time:
5 minutes
Cooking Time:
5 minutes

¾ cup tomato juice   1 tablespoon soy sauce
½ cup pineapple juice   2 teaspoons balsamic vinegar

Place all ingredients in a saucepan and cook, uncovered, stirring occasionally until slightly thickened, about 5 minutes.

Mexican Fresh Tomato Pasta Sauce

4 large ripe tomatoes, chopped
3 green onions, thinly sliced
1 4-ounce can chopped green
  chilies
¼ cup chopped cilantro

2 tablespoons lime juice
¼ teaspoon salt
freshly ground black pepper to
  taste

Servings: 4
Preparation Time:
10 minutes

Combine all ingredients in a bowl and mix well. Serve at once over cooked pasta, or let rest at room temperature until serving, up to 1 hour.

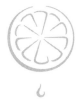

Alfredo Sauce

1 10.5-ounce package lite silken
  tofu
½ cup soy milk or water
2 tablespoons tahini
1 tablespoon soy sauce

1 tablespoon nutritional yeast
1 teaspoon minced fresh garlic
½ teaspoon onion powder
freshly ground black pepper to
  taste

Servings: 4
Preparation Time:
10 minutes
Cooking Time:
5 minutes

Combine all ingredients in a food processor and process until smooth. Pour into a saucepan and heat through, about 5 minutes. Do not boil. Serve over pasta, sprinkled with soy parmesan cheese, if desired.

Jazzy Red Pepper Sauce

Servings: makes
2 cups
Preparation Time:
10 minutes
Cooking Time:
20 minutes

4 large red bell peppers, finely
  chopped
1 large onion, finely chopped
2 teaspoons minced fresh garlic
½ cup water
1 tablespoon white wine vinegar

1 tablespoon prepared
  horseradish
¼ teaspoon crushed red pepper
¼ teaspoon white pepper
dash or two of Tabasco sauce

Use a food processor to finely chop the bell peppers and onion. Place the peppers, onion, and garlic in a saucepan with the water. Cover and cook over low heat until the peppers are very soft, about 15 minutes, adding more water if necessary. Transfer to the food processor and process until smooth. Return to the saucepan. Add the remaining ingredients. Heat over low heat for 5 minutes to blend the flavors, stirring occasionally.

Recipe Hint: This was inspired by a sauce that we enjoyed one evening at a restaurant in Old Sacramento. Mary spent the next day trying to duplicate it and came up with this wonderful sauce. We use this as a dip for pita bread, as a spread for bread or crackers, and as a sauce for pasta.

Enchilada Sauce

1 8-ounce can tomato sauce
1½ cups water
2 tablespoons cornstarch

1½ tablespoons chili powder
¼ teaspoon onion powder
⅛ teaspoon garlic powder

*Servings: makes
2½ cups
Preparation Time:
5 minutes
Cooking Time:
5 minutes*

Combine all ingredients in a saucepan until well mixed. Cook and stir over medium heat until thickened. Serve over Mexican-flavored foods.

> **Recipe Hint:** *We use this versatile sauce on burritos, tacos, tostadas, Mexican Lasagne (page 180), and enchiladas. It keeps well in the refrigerator and reheats well over low heat.*

Green Enchilada Sauce

1 7-ounce can Mexican green
   sauce
3½ cups water

4 tablespoons cornstarch
1 to 2 tablespoons chopped fresh
   cilantro

*Servings: makes
4 cups
Preparation Time:
5 minutes
Cooking Time:
10 minutes*

Combine all ingredients except the cilantro. Cook over medium heat, stirring constantly, until the mixture boils and thickens. Add the cilantro after removing from heat.

Use hot or cold. We use it on tostadas, burritos, and other Mexican-flavored foods.

WORK, SCHOOL & PLAY

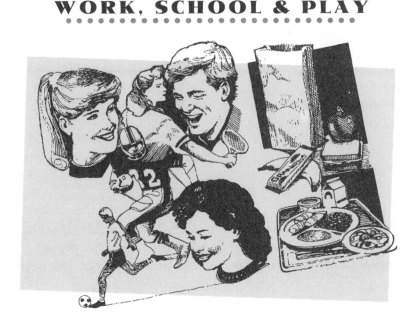

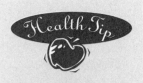

Many people complain they have no energy. Carbohydrate is the body's preferred fuel. Meat, poultry, fish, oils, and cheeses have little or no carbohydrate. No wonder so many Americans are so tired.

"*S*ack" lunches for adults and children can be made with bean and/or vegetable sandwiches. Pita bread is wonderful stuffed with canned beans and vegetables mixed with oil-free salad dressings. Pack leftovers in plastic containers. Store grain or pasta salads and soups in a thermos. Use the microwave in your workplace for reheating. Instant cup meals can be made by boiling water in the microwave and pouring it into the dry contents of the package. Add fruits, cut-up vegetables, pretzels, and healthy crackers in small sealable plastic bags.

Children should be happy about the way they eat and not feel self-conscious because they are eating different foods than most of the other children. Tell them about the good they are doing for their bodies, gentle animals, and the ecology of the planet. If your coworkers tease you about your rabbit foods, tell them to just watch as you begin to look trimmer and healthier. Whenever possible, bring enough foods to share with others so they can begin to appreciate what they're missing and will know what to do if "mad cow disease" shows up at their supermarket.

Fresh Tomato Pasta Sauce

Servings: 4
Preparation Time:
10 minutes

4 large ripe tomatoes
½ cup thinly sliced onion,
    separated into rings
¼ cup finely chopped fresh basil

½ teaspoon minced fresh garlic
¼ teaspoon salt
freshly ground black pepper to
    taste

Combine all ingredients in a bowl and mix well. Serve at once over cooked pasta or let rest at room temperature, up to 1 hour, until ready to serve.

> ***Recipe Hint:*** *This is best when made with fresh vine ripe tomatoes in the summer.*

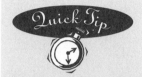

To make perfect mashed potatoes every time, drain the potatoes, reserving some of the cooking water. Mash with an electric mixer or a potato masher, adding enough cooking water to make them creamy. Do not overbeat or they will become sticky.

Mushroom Sauce

Servings: makes
2 cups
Preparation Time:
10 minutes
Cooking Time:
20 minutes

⅓ cup water
2 leeks, sliced
½ pound sliced fresh mushrooms
2 cups water
1 tablespoon soy sauce
1 teaspoon parsley flakes

½ teaspoon thyme
¼ teaspoon oregano
¼ teaspoon sage
dash or two of white pepper
2 tablespoons cornstarch mixed
    with ¼ cup cold water

Place the water, leeks, and mushrooms in a saucepan and cook, stirring frequently, for 5 minutes. Add the water and all the seasonings. Cook over low heat for 10 minutes. Slowly add the cornstarch mixture to the sauce while stirring. Cook and stir until thickened and clear, about 5 minutes. Serve over rice, potatoes, or pasta.

Asian Vegetable Mix

Servings: 4
Preparation Time:
15 minutes
Cooking Time:
10 minutes

⅓ cup water
2 tablespoons soy sauce
½ teaspoon minced fresh garlic
½ teaspoon minced fresh
  gingerroot
1 cup sliced green onions

1 cup sliced red bell pepper
1 cup broccoli florets
1 cup sliced napa cabbage
1 cup sliced fresh mushrooms
1 cup mung bean sprouts

Place the water, soy sauce, garlic, and ginger in a large nonstick frying pan. Bring to a boil. Add all the vegetables and cook, stirring occasionally, for 10 minutes.

Serve as a side dish or on top of baked potatoes, grains, or pasta.

Recipe Hint: *Buy presliced mushrooms and broccoli florets in a bag to save preparation time.*

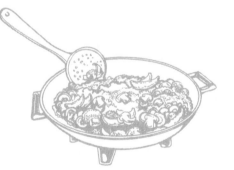

Spinach and Mushrooms

⅓ cup water
2 tablespoons soy sauce
2 tablespoons sherry
1 onion, sliced and separated
  into rings
½ pound sliced fresh mushrooms

1 6-ounce bag washed baby
  spinach
½ cup enoki mushrooms
dash of Tabasco sauce
several twists of freshly ground
  black pepper

Servings: 3
Preparation Time:
10 minutes
Cooking Time:
10 minutes

Place the water, soy sauce, and sherry in a large nonstick frying pan. Bring to a boil. Add the onion and sliced mushrooms. Cook, stirring occasionally, for 8 minutes. Add the remaining ingredients and cook, stirring frequently, until the spinach has wilted, about 2 minutes.

Serve as a side dish or on top of baked potatoes, grains, or pasta.

Recipe Hint: *Enoki mushrooms are long, thin, and white, with a very delicate taste. They are sold in bags with roots attached in the supermarket. Cut off the root, but not the stem. Use raw or cooked.*

Red Lentil Sauce

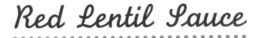

Servings: 6
Preparation Time:
5 minutes
Cooking Time:
30 minutes

4½ cups water
1 cup red lentils
1 onion, chopped
1 cup frozen chopped hash
   brown potatoes
½ cup shredded carrot

1 tablespoon soy sauce
1 teaspoon basil
¼ teaspoon dill weed
several twists of freshly ground
   black pepper

Combine all ingredients in a saucepan. Cook, uncovered, over low heat for 30 minutes, stirring occasionally.

Serve over whole wheat toast for a fast meal.

Creamy Vegetable Sauce

Servings: 4
Preparation Time:
10 minutes
Cooking Time:
20 minutes

4 cups frozen vegetables
2 cups soy or rice milk
2 tablespoons soy sauce
½ teaspoon basil

½ teaspoon dill weed
½ teaspoon ground cumin
2 tablespoons cornstarch mixed
   with ¼ cup cold water

Cook the vegetables in the milk until tender, about 15 minutes. Add the soy sauce and seasonings. Add the cornstarch mixture to the vegetable mixture while stirring. Cook and stir until thickened, about 5 minutes. Serve over whole wheat toast for a quick meal.

Recipe Hint: *Harmony Farms Fat-Free Rice Drink works well in this recipe.*

HORMONES AND DIET

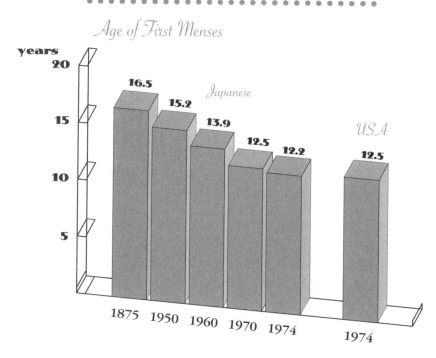

Age of First Menses

Japanese

USA

16.5	15.2	13.9	12.5	12.2		12.5
1875	1950	1960	1970	1974		1974

years
20
15
10
5

Food choices change reproductive hormone levels. For example, children mature earlier after a society changes to rich foods. In Japan, according to historical records, girls started menstruating at approximately seventeen years of age in 1875. Dietary changes in Japan following World War II resulted in earlier onset of menstruation. By 1970 Japanese girls were maturing at the same age as girls in the United States—around twelve. Boys go through a similar precocious maturity.

There are many other consequences of excess hormone stimulation from an unhealthy diet: breasts develop tenderness, lumps, and bumps—a condition called fibrocystic breast disease. The inside linings of the uterus, the endometrium, grows too thick. When this thickened endometrium sheds at the end of the month, there is a large amount of blood lost; often with cramps and blood clots. Many years of hormone overstimulation can cause dysfunctional uterine bleeding and endometrial cancer. A hysterectomy is often recommended for both conditions. The most common reason for a hysterectomy is removal of fibroid tumors, caused by years of hormone overstimulation of the uterus.

Health Tip

Many industrial chemicals dumped into our environment produce strong hormone (estrogenic) effects. These chemicals are concentrated in rich fatty foods, like meats and dairy products. The result is hormone dependent problems, like breast cancer in women and infertility in men.

Szechwan Sauce

*Servings: makes
2 cups
Preparation Time:
10 minutes
Cooking Time:
5 minutes*

1½ cups water
2 tablespoons soy sauce
⅓ cup chopped green onions
1½ tablespoons cornstarch
2 teaspoons minced fresh gingerroot

1 teaspoon minced fresh garlic
½ teaspoon Tabasco sauce
2 tablespoons chopped fresh
  cilantro (optional)

Combine all ingredients, except cilantro, in a saucepan. Cook and stir over medium heat, until the mixture boils and thickens, about 5 minutes. Add the cilantro, if desired.

Recipe Hint: *This is a very spicy sauce. Use less Tabasco and less ginger if you prefer a milder sauce. Serve over rice or other grains; use as a topping for potatoes or pasta.*

Tuscan Bean Sauce

*Servings: 4
Preparation Time:
15 minutes
Cooking Time:
10 minutes*

⅓ cup water
1 teaspoon minced fresh
  garlic
1 zucchini, quartered lengthwise,
  then sliced

1 15-ounce can white beans,
  drained and rinsed
1 14.5-ounce can chopped tomatoes
¼ cup thinly sliced fresh basil leaves
freshly ground black pepper to taste

Place the water in a saucepan. Add the garlic and zucchini. Cook, stirring occasionally, for 3 minutes. Add the beans and tomatoes. Cook for 5 minutes, stirring occasionally. Stir in the basil and pepper. Cook for 2 minutes longer.

Serve over potatoes, grains, or pasta.

Creamy Sun-Dried Tomato Sauce

3 cups sun-dried tomatoes
2 garlic cloves
2 cups boiling water

1 10.5-ounce package firm tofu
2 teaspoons light miso
dash of cayenne pepper

Place the tomatoes and garlic in a food processor or blender. Add the boiling water, cover, and let rest for 10 minutes. After 10 minutes, process briefly, then add the tofu and process until very smooth. Add the seasonings and blend again.

Serve the sauce over pasta, grains, or baked potatoes.

Recipe Hint: Be sure to buy the sun-dried tomatoes in bags, not the ones packed in oil. Check the bag to be sure they were not preserved with sulfur dioxide—many people have an allergic reaction to this substance. Cut the tomatoes with scissors.

Barbecued Tofu Sauce

1 10.5-ounce package lite silken tofu, cubed

1½ cups fat-free barbecue sauce

Place the ingredients in a nonstick frying pan and cook, stirring frequently but very gently, for 5 minutes. Serve over rice or other grains or baked potatoes.

Servings: 4
Preparation Time:
5 minutes
Resting Time:
10 minutes

Servings: 2
Preparation Time:
5 minutes
Cooking Time:
5 minutes

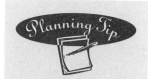

Our friend Cynthia Murata has always dedicated Sunday to preparing the week's meals for her family. She cooks and does housework at the same time. When she comes home from work during the week, dinner is only a matter of reheating.

Dilly White Sauce

*Servings: makes
2 cups
Preparation Time:
3 minutes
Cooking Time:
5 minutes*

**2 cups soy milk
2 tablespoons cornstarch
1 tablespoon soy sauce**

**1½ teaspoons dill weed
½ teaspoon ground cumin**

Combine all ingredients in a saucepan. Bring to a boil, stirring constantly, until the sauce has thickened. Serve over broccoli, asparagus, Brussels sprouts, or baked potatoes.

Onion Sauce

*Servings: makes
3 cups
Preparation Time:
5 minutes
Cooking Time:
10 minutes*

**3 cups vegetable broth
1 onion, chopped
¼ teaspoon poultry seasoning**

**4 tablespoons cornstarch mixed
with ⅓ cup cold water**

Place about ¼ cup of the vegetable broth in a saucepan. Add the onion and cook, stirring frequently, until the onion softens slightly, about 3 minutes. Add the remaining 2¾ cups vegetable broth and the poultry seasoning. Bring to a boil. Slowly add the cornstarch mixture while stirring. Cook and stir until thickened.

Serve over broccoli, cauliflower, Brussels sprouts, or baked potatoes.

INCONVENIENCE

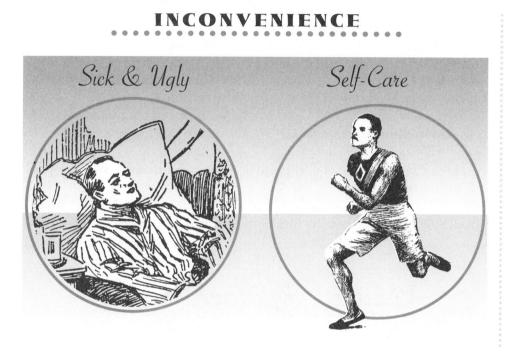

Most of us test our limits of survival daily. We smoke two packs of cigarettes, drink wine and whiskey, and consume pounds of greasy, highly processed food. And we survive! We think we are invincible. Soon, with the march of time, the hips and middle spread and the body painfully protests with headaches, bellyaches, and body aches. The doctor prescribes pills and surgeries with disturbing side effects. "I've had enough," we admit. "I'd eat cardboard to get my health back."

Knowing that you have the chance to regain lost health and appearance by eating a healthy diet, exercising, and eliminating bad habits is the first step to recovery. These three healers are more powerful than any medicines a doctor, pharmacist, or hospital can offer us. But they take effort and we procrastinate.

Finally, we change when the inconvenience of being "sick and ugly" outweighs the inconvenience of taking care of ourselves. Unfortunately, most of us learn the hard way. We wait until the elephant sits on our chest (a heart attack), or we find a lump in our breast, or the doctor insists we take blood pressure pills that destroy our sex lives. A mature person who has a high level of self-worth and knows the steps to good health will take the easy road—a healthy diet and lifestyle—long before tragedy strikes.

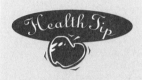

How many times have you said, "I wish I'd done that long ago." Get ahead today by carefully weighing the pain associated with bad habits and the pleasure you'll receive from good health.

Tomato-Leek Pasta Sauce

Servings: 4
Preparation Time:
10 minutes
Cooking Time:
21 minutes

⅓ cup water
3 leeks, white part only, thinly
   sliced
½ teaspoon minced fresh garlic

1 8-ounce package sliced fresh
   mushrooms
1 15-ounce can chopped tomatoes
1 8-ounce can tomato sauce

Place the water, leeks, and garlic in a large nonstick frying pan. Cook, stirring frequently, for 3 minutes. Add the mushrooms. Cook and stir for another 3 minutes. Add the tomatoes and tomato sauce. Cook, stirring occasionally, for 15 minutes. Serve over pasta.

Creamy Spinach Sauce

Servings: 6 to 8
Preparation Time:
5 minutes
Cooking Time:
10 minutes

4 cups soy milk
⅓ cup cornstarch
1 10-ounce box frozen chopped
   spinach, thawed and
   squeezed dry
1 5.5-ounce package Yves Veggie
   Pepperoni, chopped (optional)

1 tablespoon soy sauce
¼ teaspoon Worcestershire
   sauce
freshly ground black pepper to
   taste

Place the milk and cornstarch in a saucepan. Bring to a boil, whisking constantly, until thickened, about 5 minutes. Add the spinach, pepperoni, and seasonings. Cook over low heat, stirring frequently, until heated through, about 5 minutes. Serve over fat-free English muffins.

Recipe Hint: *Fat-free English muffins and crumpets are sold in most natural foods store and some supermarkets. They make great foundations for sauces or stews, or use them to make sandwiches.*

Szechwan Peanut Sauce

¼ cup peanut butter
¼ cup tahini
¼ cup rice vinegar
¼ cup soy sauce
¼ cup water

¼ teaspoon minced fresh garlic
¼ teaspoon minced fresh ginger
dash of Tabasco sauce
¼ cup roasted red peppers

Combine all ingredients, except the red pepper, in a food processor or blender. Process until smooth. Add the red pepper. Process again briefly, so flecks of red pepper pieces remain in the sauce. Use as a topping for pasta, grains, potatoes, as a spread for bread, or as a dip for vegetables. This is a very rich, high-fat sauce. Use sparingly. A little goes a long way.

Red Bean Sauce

½ cup water
1 onion, chopped
1 red bell pepper, chopped
½ teaspoon minced fresh garlic
1 15-ounce can red beans in oil-free sauce

2 tablespoons chopped canned green chilies
1 tablespoon soy sauce
1 tablespoon Worcestershire sauce
several dashes of Tabasco sauce

Place the water in a medium pot. Add the onion, bell pepper, and garlic. Cook, stirring occasionally, for 3 minutes. Add the remaining ingredients. Cook, uncovered, for about 9 minutes, stirring occasionally. Serve over potatoes, grains, or toast.

Servings: makes about 1½ cups
Preparation Time: 8 minutes

Fresh pasta made without eggs (basically semolina flour) cooks in 2 minutes in boiling water. Michelle's Natural 2 Minute Pasta (Mrs. Leepers, Inc., Poway, California) is found in most natural food stores.

Servings: 4
Preparation Time: 12 minutes
Cooking Time: 12 minutes

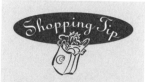

You can buy ginger and garlic ready for use in small bottles in the fresh foods section of the supermarket. Use in recipes calling for fresh garlic and gingerroot.

Hollandaise Sauce

*Servings: makes
1 cup
Preparation Time:
5 minutes
Cooking Time:
5 minutes*

¼ cup raw cashews
1 cup water
2 tablespoons lemon juice
1 teaspoon nutritional yeast
  powder
½ teaspoon onion powder
⅛ teaspoon garlic powder

⅛ teaspoon salt
¹⁄₁₆ teaspoon turmeric
pinch of paprika
1 tablespoon cornstarch mixed
  with 2 tablespoons cold water
freshly ground black pepper to
  taste

Place the cashews and ½ cup of the water in a blender. Process briefly, then gradually add the remaining water. Process until the mixture is very smooth. Pour into a saucepan. Add the lemon juice, nutritional yeast, onion powder, garlic powder, salt, turmeric, and paprika. Mix well. Add the cornstarch mixture and mix well. Bring slowly to a boil, stirring constantly, until thickened. Add the pepper to taste.

Serve over vegetables, grains, or potatoes.

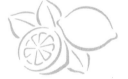

Recipe Hint: *We like this with fresh asparagus. Try the recipe for Veggie Benedicts (page 9) for a special treat.*

Asparagus and Mushroom Sauce

½ cup water
1 small onion, cut in half
   lengthwise, sliced, and
   separated into half-rings
½ pound sliced fresh mushrooms
10 stalks asparagus, sliced into
   1-inch pieces

3 cups soy or rice milk
1 tablespoon soy sauce
3 tablespoons cornstarch mixed
   with ½ cup cold water
freshly ground black pepper to
   taste

Servings: 4
Preparation Time:
10 minutes
Cooking Time:
15 minutes

Place the water in a frying pan with the onion and mushrooms. Cook, stirring frequently, for 5 minutes. Add the asparagus and cook for another 5 minutes. Add the milk and soy sauce; slowly bring to a boil. Stir in the cornstarch mixture. Cook and stir until thickened, about 5 minutes. Season with the pepper. Serve over whole wheat toast, with Oriental Wraps (page 184), or with other Asian dishes.

Recipe Hint: *Use presliced mushrooms to save time. Use other fresh vegetables in season. Cut into bite-size pieces, enough to fill 1 cup.*

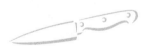

DISEASES OF "RICH" EATING

Appendicitis	*Pancreas*	**Gallstones**
Arthritis	*Prostate*	**Gastritis (ulcers)**
AS, gout,	*Testicle*	**Hemorrhoids**
psoriatic	*Uterus*	**Hiatus hernia**
rheumatoid,	**Colitis**	
Lupus	*Crohn's*	**Hypertension**
Atherosclerosis	*Ulcerative*	**Kidney failure**
Heart attacks	*Nonspecific*	**Kidney stones**
Strokes	**Constipation**	**Multiple sclerosis**
Cancers	**Diabetes**	
Colon		**Obesity**
Breast	**Diarrhea**	**Osteoporosis**
Kidney	**Diverticulosis**	**Varicose veins**

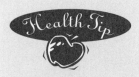

Headaches, stomachaches, arthritis, and other pains mean "something's wrong!" If you're listening, you'll change your diet and lifestyle (exercise, habits, and sleep patterns).

*T*he body fights for its survival, but years of abuse finally lead to failure of its parts and systems. What fails and when depends upon the type of injury and the body's strengths and weaknesses. A diet high in animal protein (relatively low in fat) might cause the kidneys, liver, and bones to fail early in life, while a diet high in fat and cholesterol may bring on early artery disease. Strengths and weaknesses depend upon our genetic makeup and our overall general health. Heredity is something we can't change; however, our general health can be greatly improved with a better diet and lifestyle.

Chronic diseases are better treated by diet and lifestyle changes than by taking drugs or undergoing surgery. The treatment simply stops the repeated injury caused by an unhealthy diet and lifestyle and allows the healing processes of the body to catch up. The benefits of diet and lifestyle changes for cancers is unknown but since the results of present treatment are usually so poor, any help from better self-care will greatly benefit the body.

Peppery Bean Sauce

½ cup water
1 onion, chopped
½ teaspoon minced fresh garlic
1 teaspoon dried basil
1 teaspoon dried oregano
2 zucchini, chopped

1 15-ounce can white beans
1 10-ounce jar roasted red
  peppers, coarsely chopped
1 tablespoon soy sauce
dash or two of Tabasco sauce

Place the water in a large pot. Add the onion, garlic, basil, and oregano. Cook, stirring occasionally, for 3 minutes. Add the zucchini. Cook for another 2 minutes. Add the remaining ingredients and cook for 10 minutes, stirring occasionally. Serve over pasta, grains, potatoes, or toast.

Servings: 6
Preparation Time:
15 minutes
Cooking Time:
15 minutes

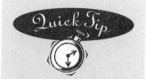

Pressure cook or boil a large pot of your favorite beans. Package them in meal-size portions in plastic bowls with covers or sealable plastic bags. Refrigerate or freeze.

Spicy Tomato Sauce

2 onions, chopped
1½ teaspoons minced fresh garlic
½ cup water
1 28-ounce can crushed tomatoes
1 10-ounce can Ro-tel diced
  tomatoes and green chilies

1 tablespoon parsley flakes
1 teaspoon dried basil
1 teaspoon dried oregano
several dashes of Tabasco
  sauce

Place the onions and garlic in a large pan with the water. Cook, stirring frequently, for 3 to 4 minutes. Add the remaining ingredients and cook for 15 minutes longer, stirring occasionally.

Servings: makes
about 5 cups
Preparation Time:
10 minutes
Cooking Time:
20 minutes

Recipe Hint: *This is a spicy alternative to Italian spaghetti sauce. It is also excellent on baked potatoes. To make this into a chunkier vegetable sauce, add some chopped green bell pepper or sliced mushrooms.*

Cynthia's Eggplant Spaghetti Sauce

Servings: 8
Preparation Time:
15 minutes
Cooking Time:
30 minutes

Both the supermarket and natural food stores carry many varieties of oil-free sauces. Use as they come over pasta or "doctor" them up with onions, green bell peppers, and mushrooms—add your favorite spices. Use sauces in soups and stews for added flavor.

⅔ cup water
1 onion, chopped
1 green or red bell pepper, chopped
1 teaspoon minced fresh garlic
2 large eggplants, chopped into bite-size pieces
1 26-ounce bottle fat-free spaghetti sauce

¼ cup red wine
1 tablespoon capers
1 teaspoon basil
1 teaspoon oregano
freshly ground black pepper to taste
pinch of crushed red pepper (optional)

Place ⅓ cup of the water into a large sauce pot. Add the onion, bell pepper, and garlic. Cook, stirring occasionally, for 5 minutes. Add the eggplant and the remaining ⅓ cup water. Cook, covered, for another 5 minutes, stirring occasionally. Add the remaining ingredients and simmer, uncovered, for 20 minutes. To make a spicier sauce, add ½ cup of medium salsa.

Hungarian Bean Sauce

Servings: 4
Preparation Time:
10 minutes
Cooking Time:
15 minutes

⅓ cup water
2 leeks, thinly sliced
1 zucchini, quartered lengthwise, then sliced
1 15-ounce can red beans, drained and rinsed

1 14.5-ounce can chopped tomatoes
¼ cup sliced roasted red peppers
1 teaspoon dried basil
½ teaspoon dried dill weed
½ teaspoon paprika

Place the water in a saucepan. Add the leeks and zucchini and cook, stirring occasionally, for 5 minutes. Add the remaining ingredients and cook, uncovered, for 10 minutes.
    Serve over potatoes or grains.

ATHEROSCLEROSIS & PLAQUE RUPTURE

Atherosclerotic plaques are filled with semiliquid, fatty, and necrotic material

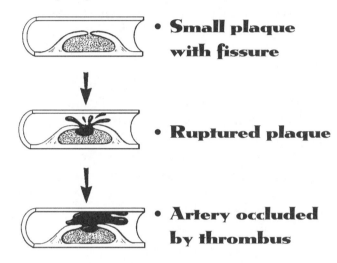

- **Small plaque with fissure**

- **Ruptured plaque**

- **Artery occluded by thrombus**

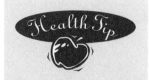

Cholesterol and triglycerides are often confused. Cholesterol is a waxy substance and triglycerides are fats—like fat on cold chicken soup. Years of eating the rich American diet cause either or both to rise in many people.

Atherosclerosis is the disease that destroys the arteries of millions of Americans every year, eventually leading to heart attacks, strokes, hearing loss, kidney failure, impotence, disability, immobility, and leg and back pain. The disease process begins when the inside linings of the arteries are injured by oxidized cholesterol, by-products of cigarette smoke combustion, and antibody reactions started by eating meat and dairy products. Slivers of cholesterol and globs of fat leak under the inside linings, causing festering sores known as atherosclerotic plaques. Your arteries contain no nerves to tell you about the ongoing damage, so you take no action until a tragedy such as a heart attack or stroke occurs.

The tragedy of complete artery closure begins with the rupture of a *tiny* overstuffed plaque. Necrotic, fatty material spurts out into the flowing blood causing the blood to clot and closing off the artery. The blood clot is called a thrombus and a heart attack is known as a coronary thrombosis.

This disease is prevented and reversed by following a low-fat, no-cholesterol, starch-based diet.

À la King Sauce

Servings: 4
Preparation Time:
15 minutes
Cooking Time:
15 minutes

½ cup water
1 onion, chopped
1 green bell pepper, chopped
½ pound sliced fresh mushrooms
½ cup unbleached white flour
3 cups soy or rice milk

1 4-ounce jar chopped pimientos
2 tablespoons soy sauce
1 teaspoon Worcestershire sauce
⅛ teaspoon white pepper
2 tablespoons cornstarch mixed
    with ¼ cup cold water

Place the water in a large pan, add the onion, green pepper, and mushrooms, and cook, stirring occasionally, for 10 minutes. Stir in the flour and continue to cook for 2 minutes, stirring constantly. Then slowly stir in the milk. Cook over medium heat, stirring almost constantly until the mixture boils, about 2 minutes. Stir in the pimientos, soy sauce, Worcestershire sauce, and pepper. Gradually add the cornstarch mixture while stirring. Cook, stirring constantly, until the mixture thickens, about 1 minute.

Serve over whole wheat toast.

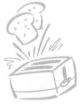

Recipe Hint: *For the past 15 years we have eaten this sauce over toasted bread or English muffins, but it would also be delicious over potatoes or grains. This version is one of the easiest and also the one we like the best.*

Summer Vegetable Sauce

½ cup water
1 onion, sliced and separated
   into rings
1 green bell pepper, thinly sliced
1 cup sliced fresh mushrooms
1 zucchini, cut in half lengthwise,
   then sliced
1 cup green beans, cut in 1-inch
   pieces
1 cup frozen corn kernels

2 fresh tomatoes, chopped
½ cup vegetable broth
2 tablespoons soy sauce
½ teaspoon dried basil
½ teaspoon dried dill weed
¼ teaspoon ground cumin
¼ teaspoon paprika
1 tablespoon cornstarch mixed
   with ¼ cup cold water

Servings: 4
Preparation Time:
15 minutes
Cooking Time:
20 minutes

Place the water in a pot with the onion and bell pepper. Cook, stirring occasionally, for 3 minutes. Add all the remaining ingredients, except the cornstarch mixture. Cook, stirring occasionally, for 15 minutes. Add the cornstarch mixture. Cook, stirring constantly until thickened, about 2 minutes.

Serve over potatoes, grains, pasta, or fat-free toast or muffins for a fast, easy summer meal.

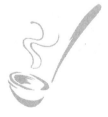

Spicy Oriental Vegetable Sauce

Servings: 4
Preparation Time:
15 minutes
Cooking Time:
10 minutes

⅓ cup water
1 onion, sliced and separated
   into rings
1 cup baby bok choy, sliced
½ pound sliced fresh mushrooms
1 cup broccoli florets
1 cup sliced asparagus
2 cups sliced napa cabbage
1 cup mung bean sprouts

¼ cup soy sauce
3 tablespoons chopped cilantro
2 tablespoons rice vinegar
1½ tablespoons cornstarch
½ teaspoon minced fresh garlic
½ teaspoon minced fresh
   gingerroot
¼ teaspoon crushed red
   pepper

Place the water in a pot with the onion, bok choy, and mushrooms. Cook, stirring occasionally, for 3 minutes. Add the broccoli, asparagus, and cabbage. Cook, stirring occasionally, for 5 minutes. Add the bean sprouts and cook for 2 minutes.

Meanwhile, combine the remaining ingredients in a bowl and mix well. Stir this mixture into the vegetables and cook and stir until thickened.

Use as a topping for grains or potatoes, or roll up in a tortilla.

Quick Tip

When stir-frying, add the vegetables to a wok with a nonstick surface on medium-high heat. Lift and turn the vegetables constantly to prevent sticking. Use oil-free liquids to sauté, such as soy sauce, nonfat salad dressing, white wine, vinegar, fruit juice, or water and herbs. After cooking the vegetables, move them up the sides of the wok to keep warm and pour the sauce into the center for thickening with cornstarch.

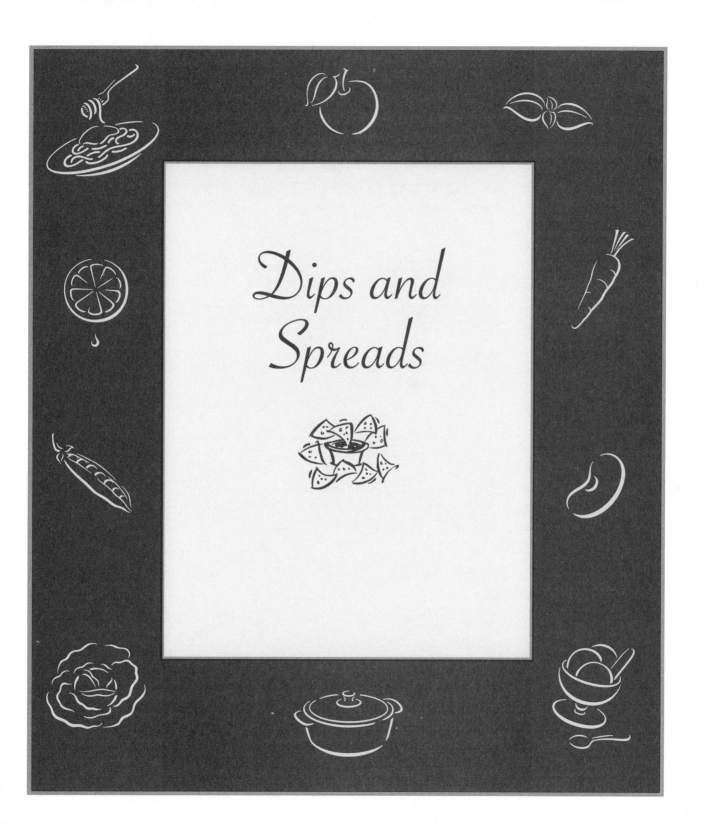

Dips and Spreads

Fiesta Black Bean Dip

2 15-ounce cans black beans,
drained and rinsed
12 ounces fresh salsa, slightly
drained

2 tablespoons tomato paste
½ teaspoon minced fresh garlic
⅛ cup fresh parsley, minced

*Servings: makes
2½ cups
Preparation Time:
5 minutes
Cooking Time:
4 minutes*

Mix all ingredients together in a microwave-safe bowl. Heat on high for 4 minutes. Stir and serve with baked fat-free tortilla chips.

Recipe Hint: *Wrap this dip in a soft burrito and garnish with some chopped green onions and alfalfa sprouts for a quick lunch.*

Chili Bean Spread

1 15-ounce can black beans,
drained and rinsed
½ teaspoon minced fresh garlic
2 tablespoons chopped onion
1½ tablespoons chopped canned
green chilies

1 tablespoon parsley flakes
1 teaspoon cider vinegar
1 teaspoon Dijon-style mustard
pinch of cayenne pepper

*Servings: makes
1½ cups
Preparation Time:
10 minutes
Chilling Time:
2 hours*

Place the beans in a bowl and mash with a bean masher. Add the remaining ingredients and mix well. Refrigerate at least 2 hours to blend the flavors. Spread on sandwiches.

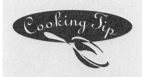

Cooking Tip

Mash cooked beans and then store them in ice cube trays or small plastic bags for later use. Add to soups, sauces, or stews for thickening and more flavor.

Deviled Spread

*Servings: makes
1½ cups
Preparation Time:
5 minutes
Chilling Time:
2 hours*

1 15-ounce can kidney beans,
  drained and rinsed
⅓ cup sweet pickle relish
¼ cup fat-free mayonnaise or
  Tofu Mayonnaise (page 255)

½ tablespoon prepared mustard
several twists of freshly ground
  black pepper

Place the beans in a medium bowl. Mash with a bean masher (do not use a food processor). Combine with the remaining ingredients. Refrigerate at least 2 hours to blend the flavors.

Use as a spread for bread, crackers, or fat-free toasted crumpets.

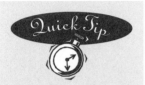

A microwave oven will turn back the clock for your flour products. Heat your breads, bagels, and tortillas on high for 15 to 45 seconds. The softness and moisture will miraculously return.

Peanut Butter Spread

*Servings: variable
Preparation Time:
5 minutes*

1 jar natural peanut butter   water

When you bring the peanut butter home from the store, let it sit undisturbed so the oil will rise to the top. Pour off as much of the oil as you are able to. Scoop out the remaining peanut butter and place in a food processor. Add about ¼ cup of water and begin to process. Slowly add more water while the machine is running. Continue to add water until the mixture is the consistency of spreadable peanut butter. Place in a jar and store in the refrigerator.

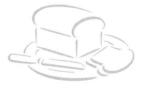

Recipe Hint: *Peanut butter is high in fat and so it is not one of our recommended foods for most adults. However, so many people have asked us for a way to make peanut butter a little healthier so they could enjoy it as a special treat once in a while. This recipe gives you the taste that you miss, with much less fat than the original. It also spreads much better. The color changes slightly after this processing.*

HEART DISEASE AND CHOLESTEROL

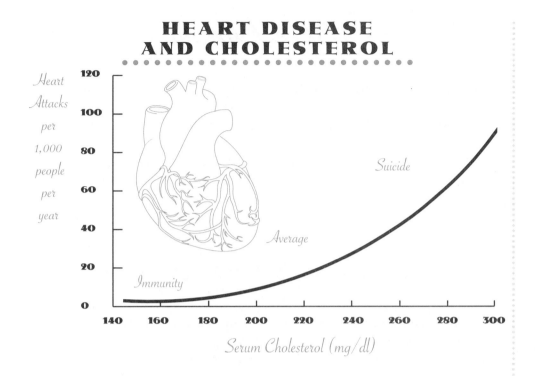

Heart Attacks per 1,000 people per year

Serum Cholesterol (mg/dl)

Immunity

Average

Suicide

*Y*our cholesterol level can be the crystal ball that predicts your chance of a heart attack and death. The average cholesterol level in the United States is about 210 mg/dl. If this is your cholesterol level, your chances of dying prematurely of a heart attack or a stroke are about 50 percent. Cholesterol levels above the 260 mg/dl range are suicidal: You are very likely to die of a complication from atherosclerosis (heart attack, stroke, or kidney failure). The ideal cholesterol level is below 150 mg/dl. Populations and individuals with cholesterol levels below 150 mg/dl have a very low risk of heart disease and are considered by some experts to be almost immune from the ravages of atherosclerosis. A cholesterol level below 150 mg/dl is a great big A+ on your health report card. People with high cholesterol should check their blood levels every one to three months.

When cholesterol rises 60 mg/dl, the risk of dying from heart disease increases by 500 percent. In some studies of reversal of atherosclerosis, people who were able to lower their cholesterol by more than 60 mg/dl were likely to show healing in their arteries and reversal of disease. The foundations to your efforts to lower your cholesterol and avoid heart disease are a low-fat, no-cholesterol diet, exercise, and healthy habits. Your second line of defense is medication.

Health Tip

There are many signs of heart disease, such as elevated cholesterol and high blood pressure. Unfortunately, medications treat mostly the signs, leaving the arteries to close down. A healthy diet treats the underlying sick arteries ... and the signs of impending doom usually come down.

Fat-Free Hummus

Servings: makes
2½ cups
Preparation Time:
5 minutes

2 15-ounce cans garbanzo beans,
   drained and rinsed
1 teaspoon minced fresh garlic

⅓ cup packed chopped parsley or
   cilantro
⅛ cup water

Place all ingredients in a food processor and process until smooth. Serve as a dip with pita bread or use as a sandwich spread.

Barbecued Garbanzo Dip

Servings: makes
1½ cups
Preparation Time:
5 minutes
Chilling Time:
2 hours

1 15-ounce can garbanzo beans,
   drained and rinsed
¼ cup diced canned green chilies

¼ cup fat-free barbecue sauce
¾ teaspoon ground cumin
½ teaspoon minced fresh garlic

Place all ingredients in a food processor and process until smooth. Use as a dip for crackers, fat-free chips, or vegetables, or as a spread for bread.

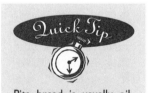

Pita bread is usually oil-free and can be found in most supermarkets. It comes in whole wheat or white varieties. Keep some in your pantry for a quick snack, or stuff with beans and vegetables for an easy meal.

Roasted Red Garbanzo Dip

1 15-ounce can garbanzo beans,
   drained and rinsed
1 7-ounce jar roasted red
   peppers, drained
½ cup plain nondairy yogurt

½ teaspoon minced fresh garlic
several twists of freshly ground
   black pepper
dash or two of Tabasco sauce

*Servings: makes
2 cups
Preparation Time:
5 minutes*

Combine all ingredients in a food processor or blender and process until smooth. Serve at once or refrigerate for later use.

Recipe Hint: *Use as a dip for fresh vegetables, crackers or rice cakes, fat-free baked tortilla chips, or as a spread for bread.*

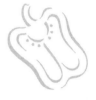

Herbed White Bean Paté

1 15-ounce can white beans,
   drained and rinsed
½ cup chopped green onions
2 tablespoons fresh parsley
1 tablespoon lemon juice
1 tablespoon tahini
1 teaspoon minced fresh garlic

1 teaspoon prepared mustard
1 teaspoon fresh finely chopped
   basil
¼ teaspoon black pepper
⅛ teaspoon nutmeg
dash of salt

*Servings: makes
2 cups
Preparation Time:
10 minutes*

Combine all ingredients in a food processor and process until blended but not completely smooth.

Place herbs in a large cup and cut with scissors into small pieces. Use 2 to 3 times as much fresh herbs as you would dry herbs.

Mock Tuna Spread

Servings: makes
2 cups
Preparation Time:
15 minutes
Chilling Time:
1 hour

1 15-ounce can garbanzo beans,
    drained and rinsed
1 stalk celery, finely chopped
¼ cup finely chopped onion

¼ cup finely chopped green onions
1 tablespoon lemon juice
¼ cup fat-free mayonnaise or
    Tofu Mayonnaise (page 255)

Place the beans in a food processor and process until coarsely chopped or mash with a bean masher. Don't overprocess to a smooth consistency.

Place in a bowl and add the remaining ingredients. Mix well. Chill at least 1 hour to blend the flavors.

Recipe Hint: *Add 2 tablespoons of pickle relish to this spread to jazz it up. We like this spread on crackers or toasted fat-free crumpets.*

Spicy Lentil Spread

Servings: makes
4 cups
Preparation Time:
5 minutes
Cooking Time:
30 minutes

2 cups red lentils
4 cups water
1 tablespoon soy sauce

1 tablespoon curry powder
½ teaspoon ground cumin

Pick over the lentils and look for stones. Place all ingredients in a medium saucepan. Bring to a boil, reduce heat, cover, and cook over low heat for 30 minutes, stirring occasionally.

Recipe Hint: *Use as a spread for bread or a filling for pita, or roll up in a tortilla. Add chopped green onion, alfalfa sprouts, chopped tomato, shredded carrots, and chopped cilantro, if desired, before eating.*

White Bean Spread

1 15-ounce can white beans,
   drained and rinsed
1 teaspoon minced fresh garlic
1 tablespoon lemon juice
½ tablespoon soy sauce

½ tablespoon balsamic vinegar
1 teaspoon Tabasco sauce
1 tablespoon chopped fresh
   cilantro or parsley
1 to 2 tablespoons water

Servings: makes
2 cups
Preparation Time:
5 minutes

Place all ingredients, except the water, in a food processor. Process until smooth. Add water as necessary to make the dip creamy.

Recipe Hint: *To make this into a chunky vegetable bean dip, add some chopped green onions and some chopped red or green bell pepper. This is wonderful as a dip for vegetables or as a sandwich spread.*

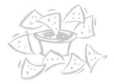

Asian Garbanzo Spread

1 15-ounce can garbanzo beans,
   drained and rinsed
2 green onions, chopped
¼ cup cilantro leaves
¼ cup orange juice
2 tablespoons rice vinegar
1 tablespoon soy sauce

1 teaspoon Dijon–style mustard
½ teaspoon minced fresh garlic
¼ teaspoon minced fresh
   gingerroot
¼ teaspoon ground coriander
¼ teaspoon ground cumin
¼ teaspoon turmeric

Servings: makes
about 2 cups
Preparation Time:
10 minutes

Place all ingredients in a food processor and process until smooth. Serve with Baked Pita Wedges (page 264). This is excellent as a dip or a spread.

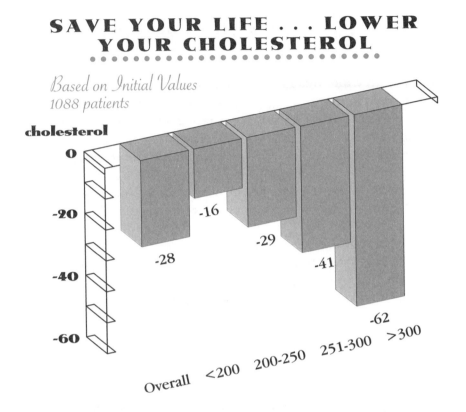

SAVE YOUR LIFE . . . LOWER YOUR CHOLESTEROL

Based on Initial Values
1088 patients

cholesterol

0

-20   -16

-28   -29

-40   -41

-62

-60

Overall   <200   200-250   251-300   >300

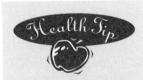

Fruit, fruit juice, honey, and other simple sugars will cause the triglycerides and cholesterol to rise in many people. Avoid these sweet tasting foods when trying to lower these blood values and your risk of heart disease.

*C*holesterol is a waxy substance made only by animals. Plants do not make or contain cholesterol. Human beings make approximately 1,000 mg of cholesterol daily, which is used to make bile acids, reproductive hormones, vitamin D, and parts of cells. We make all we require for these purposes; therefore, cholesterol is not a nutrient (a substance that must be present in our food).

Most Americans also consume 300 to 1000 mg of cholesterol daily from animal-derived foods. Unfortunately, our livers have a limited capacity to remove this excess cholesterol. As a result, the cholesterol builds up and is deposited in our blood, body fat, tendons, skin, and artery walls.

When patients at our program at St. Helena Hospital in the Napa Valley were placed on a low-fat, no-cholesterol diet, their blood cholesterol levels plummeted. In the first five days they fell 15 mg/dl. That's 3 mg each day. On the average by the 11th day they had reduced their cholesterol by 29 mg/dl. However, patients with very high cholesterol, greater than 300 mg/dl, saw their levels fall 62 mg/dl in less time than most people spend on summer vacation.

White Bean Paté

1 15-ounce can white beans, drained and rinsed
2 tablespoons vegetable broth
2 tablespoons lemon juice
1 tablespoon Dijon–style mustard
½ teaspoon minced fresh garlic
¼ teaspoon salt
⅛ teaspoon white pepper
2 tablespoons drained capers
2 tablespoons finely chopped fresh parsley or cilantro
paprika

Servings: makes 1½ cups
Preparation Time: 5 minutes

Place the beans, broth, lemon juice, mustard, garlic, salt, and pepper into a food processor or blender and process until smooth. Place in a bowl and stir in the capers and parsley or cilantro. Sprinkle the paprika over the top to garnish.

Recipe Hint: *Serve as a spread for crackers or rice cakes, Baked Pita Wedges (page 264), or sandwiches. Use as a dip for raw vegetables.*

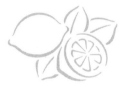

Sweet Bean Spread

1 15-ounce can kidney beans, drained and rinsed
⅓ cup Peanut Butter Spread (recipe page 246)
3 teaspoons honey
1½ teaspoons vanilla
¾ teaspoon cinnamon

Servings: makes 1½ cups
Preparation Time: 5 minutes

Place all ingredients in a food processor and process until well mixed, but not completely pureed. Serve as a dip for vegetables, or spread on bread, crackers, or rice cakes.

Recipe Hint: *Our office staff introduced us to this spread. They like to dip sticks of jicama in it.*

Black Bean Dip

Servings: makes
1½ cups
Preparation Time:
5 minutes

Servings: makes
2½ cups
Preparation Time:
5 minutes

1 16-ounce can black beans,
  drained and rinsed
½ cup salsa

3 tablespoons cilantro leaves
2 tablespoons lime juice
½ teaspoon ground cumin

Combine all ingredients in a food processor and process until smooth. Serve with fat-free tortilla chips.

Recipe Hint: *Stack several whole wheat or corn tortillas. Cut across the middle to make 6 to 10 wedges. Heat on a baking sheet in the oven for 10 minutes.*

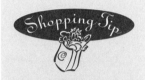

Precooked and even non-fat refried beans can be found in every super-market. There are black, white, red, kidney, and pinto beans. Use them for "almost instant burritos and tortillas" made by spreading whole or mashed beans on a corn or whole wheat tortilla and adding tomatoes, onions, sprouts, and your favorite salsa. Use cooked whole beans for the foundation of cold salads or add them to soups and stews.

Pinto Bean Dip

1 16-ounce can fat-free refried
  beans
5 ounces lite silken tofu
¾ cup salsa

1 teaspoon minced fresh
  garlic
1 teaspoon chili powder
2 to 3 green onions, chopped

Place all ingredients, except the green onions, in a food processor. Process until smooth. Place in a bowl and stir in the green onions. Serve with fat-free tortilla chips.

Red Pepper Dip

1 16-ounce package fresh tofu, drained
2 tablespoons lemon juice
1 tablespoon cider vinegar
⅓ cup canned roasted red peppers

1 teaspoon chili powder
several dashes of Tabasco sauce
¼ teaspoon salt (optional)

Servings: makes 2 cups
Preparation Time: 10 minutes

Combine the tofu, lemon juice, and vinegar in a food processor. Process until smooth. Add the peppers and chili powder. Process for several minutes until very smooth and creamy. Add Tabasco and salt.

Recipe Hint: Roasted red peppers are sold in bottles in the supermarket. This dip keeps well in the refrigerator for several days, if it lasts that long in your house! Use as a dip for raw vegetables or fat-free chips. Use as a spread for crackers or bread. Also good on baked potatoes.

Tofu Mayonnaise

Servings: makes 1⅓ cups
Preparation Time: 5 minutes

1 10.5-ounce package lite silken tofu
1½ tablespoons lemon juice
1 teaspoon honey

½ teaspoon salt
½ teaspoon dry mustard
⅛ teaspoon white pepper

Place all ingredients in a blender jar and process until smooth and creamy.

Recipe Hint: Use Tofu Mayonnaise in sandwiches, salads, and spreads.

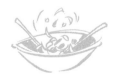

FAMILIAR FOODS

Breakfast	Lunch	Dinner	Dessert
Oatmeal	Bean soup	Manicotti	Apple crisp
Corn flakes	Gazpacho	Spaghetti	Carrot cake
Pancakes	Sandwich	Burritos	Pumpkin pie
Waffles	Fast pizza	Enchiladas	Peach pie
Hash browns	Burgers	Spanish rice	Fruit
Grits	Sloppy joe	Stew	Sorbet
Bagels	Tostada	Chop suey	Banana bread
Breads	Pasta salad	Moo shu	Oatmeal cookies
Fruit	Potato salad	Cabbage rolls	Cinnamon buns
Smoothies	Green salad	Ratatouille	Rice pudding

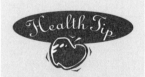

Simple diets provide excellent nutrition. Throughout history people didn't worry about eating a "well balanced diet," rather, they hoped only for enough rice or potatoes to feed the family. Look around you to see the consequences of eating a wide variety of foods—obesity and disease.

*Y*our goal is to find about a dozen dishes you enjoy. You have your favorites right now. You probably have the same thing for breakfast every day. For lunch you choose between a couple of items and dinner is a matter of selecting among four or five favorites. When you go out to eat you probably always order the same item from the menu at that particular restaurant. People are rather monotonous in their eating habits. Since there are more than 1700 recipes in the McDougall books, finding new favorites will be an enjoyable adventure.

You have spent many years learning to cook the American diet and adjusting to its tastes, therefore it should not surprise you that a change to a healthier way of eating may take some time and effort. Pick one or two recipes from this book that seem to be good possibilities because they look interesting and have ingredients and spices you have enjoyed in other recipes. Don't go overboard by making a multi-course meal, as you did when you cooked the "well-balanced" American diet. Prepare the new recipes several times over the next month—they will soon become your favorites.

Spinach Dip

1 10-ounce box frozen chopped
  spinach, thawed and squeezed
  dry
1 bunch green onions, chopped
1 pound tofu
2 tablespoons lemon juice

2 teaspoons dill weed
1½ teaspoons honey
¾ teaspoon dry mustard
¼ teaspoon salt
¼ teaspoon white pepper

*Servings: makes
3 cups
Preparation Time:
10 minutes
Chilling Time:
2 hours*

Place the spinach and green onions in a bowl. Place the remaining ingredients in a blender or food processor and process until smooth. Add to the spinach and green onions and mix well. Refrigerate to blend the flavors. Use as a dip for bread, crackers, or vegetables. Try this on baked potatoes, too.

Recipe Hint: *To make a smooth, creamy green dip, place all ingredients in food processor and process until smooth.*

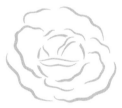

Tofu Sour Cream

1 10.5-ounce package lite silken
  tofu
2 tablespoons lemon juice

2 teaspoons sugar
pinch salt

*Servings: makes
1 ¼ cups
Preparation Time:
5 minutes
Chilling Time:
2 hours*

Combine all ingredients in a food processor and process until smooth. Refrigerate at least 2 hours to blend the flavors. Use any time you would use dairy sour cream.

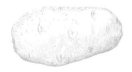

Curry Tofu Dip

Servings: makes
1¼ cups
Preparation Time:
5 minutes
Chilling Time:
1 hour

1 10.5-ounce package firm lite silken tofu
1½ teaspoons curry powder

1 tablespoon parsley flakes
⅛ teaspoon salt (optional)

Combine all ingredients in a blender jar and process until smooth.

Recipe Hint: This is a wonderful dip for raw vegetables. It is also one of my favorite dips for artichoke leaves. Prepare the artichokes by cutting off the stems. Remove the loose outer leaves and cut off the tops. Use scissors to snip off the tops of sharp leaves. Cook in boiling water with 1 to 2 tablespoons lemon juice added for about 45 minutes. After cooking, pull out the center leaves and remove the fuzzy centers with a spoon. Also try this dip with asparagus and baked potatoes.

Chickenless Salad

Servings: makes
1½ cups
Preparation Time:
10 minutes

1 10.5-ounce package lite silken tofu
¼ cup fat-free mayonnaise or Tofu Mayonnaise (page 255)
⅛ cup chopped green onions
⅛ cup finely chopped celery
⅛ cup sweet pickle relish

1 tablespoon prepared mustard
1 tablespoon soy sauce
¼ teaspoon garlic powder
¼ teaspoon turmeric
several twists of freshly ground black pepper

Mash the tofu with a bean masher. Combine with the remaining ingredients in a bowl. Serve at once or refrigerate until serving.

Recipe Hint: This makes an excellent spread for bread, crackers, pita, crumpets, or vegetables.

Eggless Egg Salad

1 10.5-ounce package lite silken tofu
¼ cup finely chopped celery
¼ cup fat-free mayonnaise or Tofu Mayonnaise (page 255)
⅛ cup finely chopped onion
2 teaspoons vinegar

2 teaspoons dried chives
½ teaspoon turmeric
¼ teaspoon onion powder
¼ teaspoon garlic powder
¼ teaspoon dill weed
¼ teaspoon salt (optional)

Place the tofu in a medium bowl. Mash with a fork or bean masher until finely crumbled but not smooth. Add the remaining ingredients and mix well. Chill at least 2 hours before serving to attain the best flavor and bright yellow color.

Fresh Salsa

1 15-ounce can chopped tomatoes
⅓ cup chopped onion
1 4-ounce can chopped green chilies

¼ cup finely chopped fresh cilantro
1 tablespoon fresh lime juice
¼ teaspoon salt
dash or two of Tabasco sauce

Place all ingredients in a food processor or blender and process briefly until just blended.

Recipe Hint: *This salsa is inspired by one served at our favorite Mexican restaurant in Hawaii, Bueno Nalo. Use it as a topping for burritos or other Mexican–style food, or serve it as a dip for oven-baked tortilla chips (Recipe Hint page 254) or raw vegetables. It will keep in the refrigerator for about 1 week.*

Servings: makes
1½ cups
Preparation Time:
10 minutes
Chilling Time:
2 hours

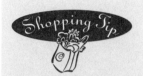

Tofu is sold both fresh and aseptically packaged. Fresh tofu usually comes in 1-pound packages and is found in the refrigerated section. Drain before using. Aseptically packaged tofu is 10.5 ounces and may be sold cold or at room temperature. Both kinds have an expiration date on the package.

Servings: makes
2 cups
Preparation Time:
10 minutes

Nutty Soft Taco Filling

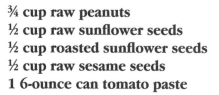

Servings: makes
2½ cups
Preparation Time:
15 minutes
Cooking Time:
30 minutes

¾ **cup raw peanuts**
½ **cup raw sunflower seeds**
½ **cup roasted sunflower seeds**
½ **cup raw sesame seeds**
1 6-ounce can tomato paste

1 teaspoon ground cumin
1 teaspoon soy sauce
½ **teaspoon chili powder**
¼ **teaspoon onion powder**
⅛ **teaspoon garlic powder**

Place the peanuts and raw sunflower seeds in a saucepan with water to cover. Cook, covered, over medium heat for 30 minutes. Remove from heat and drain; reserve the cooking liquid. Place the cooked nuts in a food processor with the roasted sunflower seeds and the sesame seeds. Process briefly. Add the tomato paste and process again. Add enough water to the reserved cooking liquid to make 1 cup. Gradually add the liquid to the nut mixture while processing. Add the seasonings. Process until well blended.

> ***Recipe Hint:*** *Use this rich, high-fat, tasty filling in soft corn tortillas. Top with chopped green onions, chopped tomatoes, alfalfa sprouts, and salsa.*

EVOLUTION OF
FOOD RECOMMENDATIONS

1·basic 4   *2·pyramid*

3·McDougall Trapezoid

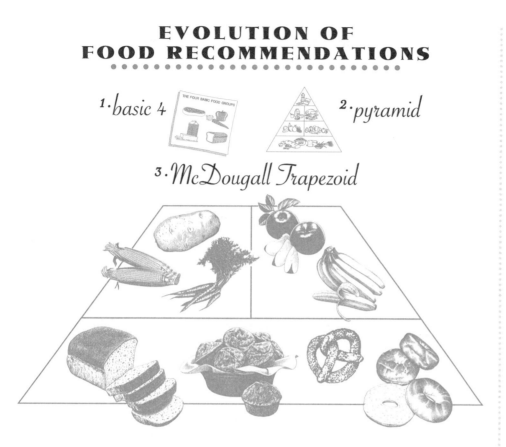

We were all raised with the "Four Basic Food Groups"—a concept that allowed us to eat anything and everything that would fit between our lips. This thinking was founded on the idea that people suffer disease as a result of deficiencies. However, "deficiency" diseases are not our problem. It's likely you never met anyone with beriberi, pellagra, or scurvy. On the other hand, you probably have many friends and relatives who suffer from diseases caused by excess fat, salt, cholesterol, and animal protein in their diets.

The U.S. Department of Agriculture recently developed the "Food Guide Pyramid," which reduced the Four Basic Food Groups' recommended amount of meat, dairy products, eggs, oils, and refined foods, and instead encouraged the use of more whole grains, fresh fruits, and vegetables. The evolution of recommendations for eating for good health will be complete when the country adopts "The McDougall Food Trapezoid," which simply chops off the unhealthy top of the food pyramid.

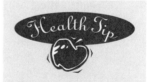

People are learning the truth about good eating. Soon shoveling high fat, greasy foods into one's body will be viewed as disgusting as smoking cigarettes is today. The American diet is a dangerous fad, now being replaced by sensible eating.

Bean Guacamole

Servings: makes
2½ cups
Preparation Time:
5 minutes

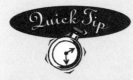

Quick Tip

Avocados discolor when exposed to air. To keep mashed avocado looking fresh longer, place the pit in the bowl and cover with plastic wrap.

1 15-ounce can white beans, drained and rinsed
1 small avocado, mashed
½ cup mild salsa
¼ cup finely chopped green onions

2 tablespoons canned chopped green chilies
2 tablespoons chopped cilantro
1 tablespoon lemon juice
½ teaspoon minced fresh garlic
¼ teaspoon salt

Mash the beans with a bean or potato masher. Combine all ingredients in a bowl and mix well. Serve with baked fat-free tortilla chips.

Surprise Vegetable Salsa

Servings: makes
2 cups
Preparation Time:
10 minutes
Chilling Time:
2 hours

1 cup finely chopped cucumber
½ cup chopped green onions
½ cup finely chopped red bell pepper
⅓ cup chopped fresh cilantro

½ teaspoon minced fresh garlic
2 tablespoons soy sauce
1 tablespoon rice vinegar
¼ teaspoon crushed red pepper
dash of sesame oil (optional)

Combine all ingredients in a medium bowl and refrigerate at least 2 hours to blend the flavors.

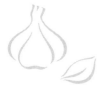

Recipe Hint: Use this salsa as a dip for fresh vegetables or try with fat-free baked tortilla chips or Baked Pita Wedges (page 264).

Black Bean and Corn Salsa

1 15-ounce can black beans,
   drained and rinsed
2 tomatoes, chopped
¾ cup frozen corn kernels, thawed
4 green onions, chopped
2 tablespoons chopped and
   canned green chilies

2 tablespoons chopped fresh
   cilantro
¼ cup lemon juice
½ teaspoon ground cumin
several twists of freshly ground
   black pepper
½ cup diced avocado (optional)

*Servings: makes
3 cups
Preparation Time:
10 minutes*

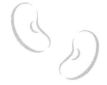

Combine all ingredients, except avocado, in a bowl. Mix well. Stir in avocado, if desired. Serve at once.

Recipe Hint: *If you are not going to serve this salsa immediately, do not add the avocado until just before serving because it will discolor.*

Radish Salsa

*Servings: makes
1½ cups
Preparation Time:
15 minutes
Chilling Time:
30 minutes*

2 garlic cloves
**1 very small serrano chili
    (optional)**
4 bunches radishes, cleaned
2 large tomatoes, cut in quarters

½ cup cilantro
⅛ teaspoon salt
**freshly ground black pepper to
    taste**

Mince the garlic and chili in a food processor. Add the radishes and process just until coarsely chopped. Add the tomatoes and cilantro and process until the salsa is the desired consistency. Add the salt and pepper. Cover and chill for at least 30 minutes. Serve with tortilla chips.

Baked Pita Wedges

*Servings: variable
Preparation Time:
5 minutes
Cooking Time:
20 to 30 minutes*

6 loaves pita bread

Preheat the oven to 300 degrees.
Cut the pita bread into wedges and separate one side from the other. Place in a single layer on a baking sheet. Bake for 20 to 30 minutes until crisp. Store in an airtight container.

> *Recipe Hint: Sprinkle the wedges with some onion powder, garlic powder, chili powder, or poultry seasoning before baking for an interesting flavor.*

Planning Tip

Stock your home with only healthy foods. This will cut down on temptation. Make sure there are plenty of delicious foods available. No one can stick to a diet with unappealing dishes and no easily accessible snacks.

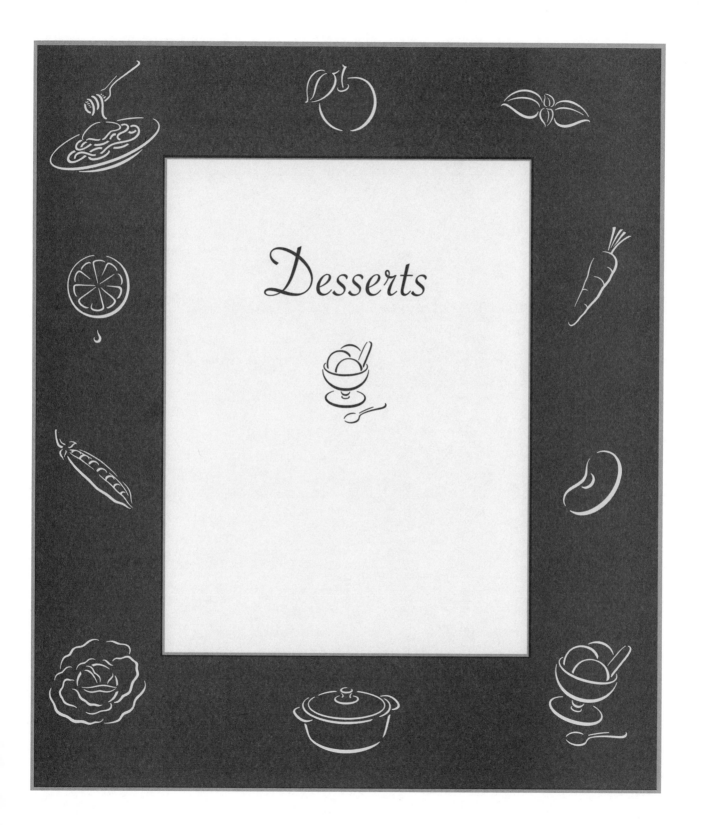

Desserts

Frozen Banana Smoothies

1 cup frozen banana chunks
¼ cup frozen fruit (strawberries, raspberries, blueberries, etc.)

1 cup fruit juice (orange, pineapple, apple, etc.)

Servings: 2
Preparation Time:
5 minutes

Place all ingredients in a blender jar and process until smooth for a "better than ice cream" frozen smoothie.

Recipe Hint: *To freeze bananas, peel, slice into chunks, freeze on a baking sheet, then store in a covered container in the freezer.*

Tofu Berry Smoothies

1 10.5-ounce package lite silken tofu
1 cup fresh berries
½ cup fruit juice

1 tablespoon honey
1 tablespoon lemon juice
1 cup ice cubes

Servings: 2
Preparation Time:
5 minutes

Place all ingredients in a blender jar and process until smooth.

Recipe Hint: *Try strawberries, raspberries, or blueberries and more exotic juices like guava, pear, or passion fruit.*

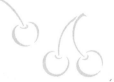

GREAT BEVERAGES
ALL VEGETABLE PRODUCTS

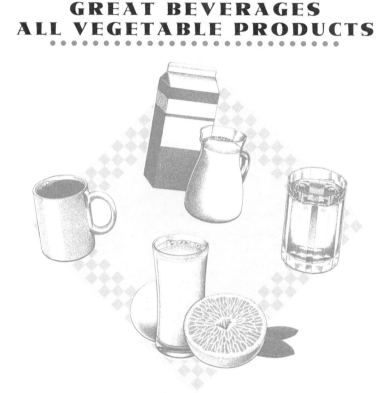

Although water fills the stomach and helps to satisfy hunger, it also speeds up the rate at which the food leaves the stomach, so you'll soon be hungry again. Drinking water before, during, or after meals does not affect weight loss.

*Y*our ideal beverage is plain pure water drunk cold, lukewarm, or hot before, during, and after your meals. And you can drink to your thirst's content. Carbonation of water makes it more flavorful for some people, but the gas causes burping, bloating, and flatus.

Herb teas taste great hot or cold. They offer mild pharmacological benefits: For example, peppermint soothes the stomach. Strong caffeinated teas stimulate. Green tea contains caffeine and is an antioxidant; drinking it may reduce your risk of heart disease. Beverages made from cereal grains, such as Postum, Cafix, Kaffree Roma, or Pero, can replace coffee.

Juices provide plenty of sweet-tasting calories and nutrients. When whole fruit or vegetables are processed in a juicer, all of the nutrients are retained, but slicing a thousand times with a steel blade adversely affects their physical properties. Drinking juice encourages weight gain and raises cholesterol and triglyceride levels in sensitive people; however, for most healthy people, especially those who need extra calories, such as children and athletes, juice makes a fine beverage.

Dreamsicles

1 10.5 ounce package lite soft
   silken tofu
1 12-ounce container frozen
   orange juice

1 cup soy milk
1 teaspoon vanilla

Servings: 6 to 8
Preparation Time:
5 minutes
Freezing Time:
4 hours

Place all ingredients in a blender jar and process until smooth.
Pour into molds and freeze for at least 4 hours.

Easy Fruit Tart

1 slice fat-free raisin-walnut
   bread

¼ cup canned fruit pie filling
   cinnamon

Servings: 1
Preparation Time:
2 minutes
Cooking Time:
30 seconds

Place the bread on a microwave-safe plate. Spoon the pie filling
over the top and sprinkle with cinnamon. Microwave on high for 30
seconds.

*Recipe Hint: Canned pie fillings are available in natural
food stores and supermarkets. Most of them contain some
simple sugar, but they do not contain any fat.*

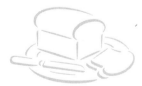

Rice Pudding

Servings: 2
Preparation Time:
5 minutes
(need cooked rice)
Cooking Time:
5 minutes

1 cup cooked brown rice
¼ cup soy milk
¼ cup fresh or dried chopped
   fruit

2 teaspoons raw sugar
½ teaspoon vanilla

Combine all ingredients in a microwave-safe bowl. Microwave on high for 5 minutes. Stir. Let stand until the soy milk is absorbed. Serve warm or cold.

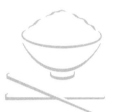

Couscous Pudding

Servings: 6
Preparation Time:
5 minutes
Cooking Time:
5 minutes
Resting Time:
15 minutes

2 cups water
¾ cup chopped dates
3 cups rice milk
¼ cup honey

1 cinnamon stick
1 cup couscous
1 teaspoon vanilla
½ teaspoon ground cinnamon

Bring the water to a boil in a small saucepan. Add the dates, cover, and set aside.

In a separate saucepan, heat the rice milk, honey, and cinnamon stick until almost boiling. Remove from heat and stir in the couscous and vanilla. Cover and let rest for 15 minutes. Remove the cinnamon stick. Drain the dates in a colander and add to the couscous. Sprinkle with cinnamon before serving.

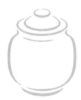

Microwaved Baked Apples

2 large cooking apples
2 tablespoons brown sugar

1 tablespoon raisins

Servings: 2
Preparation Time:
8 minutes
Cooking Time:
8 minutes
Resting Time:
5 minutes

Peel the apples halfway down and core about three quarters of the way down. Combine the brown sugar and raisins in a small bowl. Pack the brown sugar mixture into the cored apples. Place in microwave-safe bowls, cover, and cook on 70 percent power for 8 minutes, turning once halfway through the cooking time. Remove from the microwave and let rest for 5 minutes before serving.

Fruit Enchiladas

12 large strawberries, diced
1 8-ounce can crushed pineapple, drained (reserve juice)
1 cup fresh or frozen blueberries
1 cup raisins or chopped dates
1 15-ounce can pears, drained (reserve juice) and diced

1 cup unsweetened applesauce
1 teaspoon cinnamon
½ teaspoon nutmeg
½ teaspoon honey
8 fat-free flour or corn tortillas

Servings: 8
Preparation Time:
10 minutes
Cooking Time:
5 minutes

Mix the strawberries, pineapple, blueberries, and raisins or dates in a bowl. Set aside. Place the pears and ½ cup of the combined reserved juices in a saucepan. Mash with a fork or bean masher. Add the applesauce, cinnamon, nutmeg, and honey and heat over low heat until warmed through. Do not boil.

Place ½ cup of the fruit mixture down the center of each tortilla. Roll up, pour a little of the sauce over each tortilla, and serve.

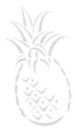

Brownies

Servings: 16
Preparation Time:
15 minutes
Cooking Time:
30 minutes

Dry ingredients:

1 cup unbleached flour
⅔ cup reduced-fat cocoa
  powder

1 teaspoon baking powder
1 teaspoon baking soda
¼ teaspoon salt

Wet ingredients:

1 cup Just Like Shortenin' or
  Wonderslim or Prune Puree
  (page 281)
1 cup sugar

1 teaspoon vanilla
2 tablespoons Egg Replacer
  mixed in ½ cup water

Preheat the oven to 350 degrees.

Combine dry ingredients in a bowl. Set aside.

Mix Just Like Shortenin' or Wonderslim or Prune Puree and sugar together in a separate bowl. Stir in the vanilla. Mix the Egg Replacer and water together and whisk until very frothy. Add to the sugar mixture and stir to combine. Add the wet ingredients to the dry ingredients and stir until mixed. Do not overmix. Spoon into a nonstick 8-inch-square baking dish and flatten. Bake for 30 minutes.

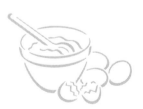

Recipe Hint: *Just Like Shortenin' is a fairly new fat replacer. It is made from plums and apples and is an excellent fat replacer in baked goods. If you cannot find it in your natural food store, information on where to purchase it may be obtained from The Plumlife Company, 15 Orchard Park, Madison, CT 06443.*

BAKING WITHOUT OIL

Carbonated Water
Applesauce
Mashed Bananas
Mashed Potatoes
Silken Tofu
Wonderslim
Pureed Prunes
Baby Food

Oil performs two functions in baking: It prevents the baked good from sticking to the pan and softens it. Nonstick silicone-coated muffin tins and bread pans will prevent sticking. Parchment paper (found in the grocery store next to the wax paper) can be used to line baking pans. Mary also places it over dishes before covering them with aluminum foil to keeping the food from coming into contact with the aluminum.

Softening is tastefully accomplished by replacing oil with applesauce, mashed bananas, baby food, or mashed potatoes. Use half of the amount of oil called for. Silken tofu can replace oil, but tofu is also high in fat (54 percent); even lite tofu is 33 percent fat. Use half as much tofu as you would oil.

Pureed prunes are an excellent oil substitute. There is a recipe for Prune Puree on page 281. Use half of the amount of oil called for. Lighter Bake, Wonderslim, Just Like Shortenin', and Lekvar are bottled ready-to-use fat replacers made from plums or prunes and are sold in your grocery or natural food store.

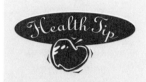

Health Tip

Gallbladder disease is found in 40 percent of people over the age of sixty. Vegetable oils promote gallbladder disease more than animal fats. Changing to a healthy, low-fat diet can prevent gallstones and often relieves the pain of gallbladder disease.

Fat-Free Fudge

Servings: 2
Preparation Time:
5 minutes
Cooking Time:
1½ minutes
Resting Time:
2 minutes

3 tablespoons low-fat soy milk
3 tablespoons carob powder
6 tablespoons sugar

1 teaspoon cream of tartar
½ teaspoon vanilla
dash of salt

Combine all ingredients in a microwave-safe bowl. Microwave on high for 60 seconds. Stir, let rest for 30 seconds, microwave on high for 10 seconds, let rest for 30 seconds; repeat the 10- and 30-second cycle two more times. Let cool and enjoy.

Recipe Hint: *Use reduced-fat cocoa powder to make this fudge taste even more familiar.*

Chocolate Fruit Fondue

Servings: 4
Preparation Time:
15 minutes
Cooking Time:
5 minutes

2 tablespoons Wonderslim cocoa
   powder
1 tablespoon cornstarch
¼ cup water

1 12-ounce can apple juice
   concentrate, thawed
2 teaspoons vanilla
4 cups mixed fresh fruit, cut into
   chunks

Combine the cocoa powder and cornstarch in a saucepan. Slowly add the water while stirring to make a smooth paste. Stir in the apple juice concentrate and vanilla. Cook over low heat, stirring constantly, until thickened, about 5 minutes. Transfer to a fondue pot or chafing dish to keep warm. Dip pieces of fruit into the warm sauce.

Recipe Hint: *Use a variety of fruit, such as strawberries, bananas, apples, mangoes, papaya, or melons. We very often serve this when we have guests. It is fun to sit around the fondue pot after dinner, dunking chunks of fresh fruit into chocolate sauce.*

Apricot Bars

. . . .

1 cup unbleached white
  flour
½ cup packed brown sugar
½ teaspoon baking powder
¼ teaspoon baking soda
⅛ teaspoon ground cloves
½ cup apricot nectar

⅓ cup Lighter Bake or
  Wonderslim or Prune Puree
  (page 281)
1 teaspoon Egg Replacer mixed in
  2 tablespoons water
½ cup finely chopped dried
  apricots

*Servings: makes
18 bars
Preparation Time:
15 minutes
Cooking Time:
25 minutes*

Preheat the oven to 350 degrees.

Combine the dry ingredients in a large bowl. Set aside.

Place the nectar and Lighter Bake or Wonderslim or Prune Puree in another bowl. Beat the Egg Replacer and water until it is very frothy, then add to the other wet ingredients and mix well. Add to the dry ingredients, stirring until just combined. Stir in the dried apricots.

Spread the batter in a nonstick 11 × 7-inch baking pan. Bake for 25 minutes or until a toothpick inserted in the center comes out clean. Cool and cut into bars.

Recipe Hint: *Lighter Bake is a new fat replacer from Sunsweet Growers. It is made from plums and apples and is an excellent fat replacer in baked goods. It should be available in most supermarkets in the baking ingredients aisle.*

Chocolate Cream Filling

Servings: 8
Preparation Time:
10 minutes
Chilling Time:
4 hours

2 10.5-ounce packages lite silken tofu
½ cup Wonderslim Low-Fat Cocoa Powder
¾ cup honey
3 teaspoons vanilla

Place the tofu in a food processor and process until very smooth. Place the cocoa in a separate bowl. Set aside.

Heat the honey in a microwave for 1½ minutes. Pour over the cocoa powder and mix until very smooth. Add the cocoa mixture and vanilla to the tofu and process again until very smooth. Pour into a baked pie crust and refrigerate for at least 4 hours.

Recipe Hint: *This is also delicious as a pudding. Pour into individual bowls and refrigerate before serving.*

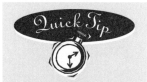

Use a large fat-free flour tortilla shell for a pie crust. Place in a pie pan and microwave for 30 seconds until soft. Press down in the pan. Fill with any pie filling. Bake as directed.

Pumpkin Pie

Servings: 8
Preparation Time:
15 minutes
Cooking Time:
1 hour
Chilling Time:
2 hours

15 ounces lite silken tofu
1 16-ounce can solid-pack pumpkin
⅔ cup honey
1 teaspoon vanilla
1 teaspoon ground cinnamon
1 teaspoon pumpkin pie spice
½ teaspoon ground ginger
¼ teaspoon ground cloves
1 pie crust (see page 279)

Preheat the oven to 350 degrees.

Combine all ingredients in a food processor and process until very smooth. Pour into a pie crust and bake for 1 hour. Remove from the oven and chill for at least 2 hours before serving.

Blueberry Pie

Crust:

1½ cups Grape Nuts cereal
¾ cup thawed unsweetened apple
  juice concentrate

½ teaspoon vanilla

Servings: 8
Preparation Time:
15 minutes
Cooking Time:
18 minutes

Filling:

1 8-ounce can unsweetened
  crushed pineapple, undrained
½ cup thawed unsweetened grape
  juice concentrate

½ cup thawed unsweetened apple
  juice concentrate
¼ cup quick-cooking tapioca
5 cups fresh or frozen blueberries

Preheat the oven to 350 degrees.

To make the crust, place the cereal in a blender or food processor and process briefly until slightly crushed. Combine the apple juice concentrate and vanilla. Mix the cereal and apple juice mixture together. Press into the bottom and sides of a 10-inch pie pan. Bake for 12 minutes. Cool.

Meanwhile, to make the filling, place the pineapple, juices, and tapioca in a medium saucepan. Bring to a boil. Cook and stir until thickened, about 3 minutes. Add the blueberries. Cook an additional 3 minutes. Pour into the crust. Cool and serve.

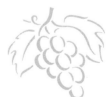

MOOD MANAGEMENT

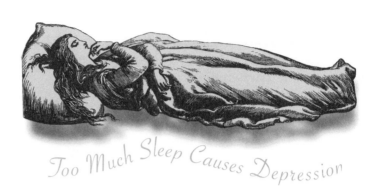

Too Much Sleep Causes Depression

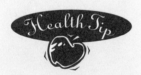

Health Tip

Most of us have been taught that sleep is good for us—the more the better—a minimum of eight hours. While children, sick people, and pregnant women may need this amount of sleep and more, most adults function best with five to seven hours.

Have you ever noticed that you felt sleepy, sluggish, or downright depressed after a "good" night's sleep—maybe eight to ten hours' worth? Something about sleep causes depression, and staying awake washes this depressogenic factor out of the system. About seventy-seven percent of people diagnosed with serious endogenous depression respond to less sleep. The right amount of sleep can be determined by trial and error—balancing fatigue which needs to be alleviated by rest and your mood which can be depressed by too much sleep.

There are three other powerful alternatives to doctor prescribed drugs to relieve depression. Exercise relieves mild depression and anxiety by producing endorphins in the nervous system. A healthy, low-animal-protein diet allows the production of neurochemicals, like serotonin, that elevate mood. Extracts of a plant, Hypercium perforatum, commonly called St. John's wort, have at least 10 compounds that may provide mood elevating effects. Two to four weeks are required to develop mood elevating effects.

Baked Apple Pie

5 cups sliced apples
⅓ cup thawed unsweetened apple
   juice concentrate
1 teaspoon cinnamon
½ teaspoon nutmeg

½ cup flour
½ cup thawed orange juice
   concentrate
1 tablespoon maple syrup
½ teaspoon baking powder

Servings: 6 to 8
Preparation Time:
15 minutes
Cooking Time:
45 minutes

Preheat the oven to 350 degrees.

Place the apples, apple juice, cinnamon, and nutmeg in a medium saucepan. Bring to a boil and cook over medium heat for 5 minutes, stirring occasionally. Remove from heat and pour into a pie plate.

Combine the remaining ingredients in a separate bowl. Crumble over the apples. Bake for 40 minutes.

Easy Pie Crust

1½ cups fat-free cookie crumbs
   or fat-free graham cracker
   crumbs

3 tablespoons thawed and
   unsweetened apple juice
   concentrate

Servings: makes
1 9-inch pie crust
Preparation Time:
5 minutes
Cooking Time:
5 minutes

Preheat the oven to 350 degrees.

Combine the crumbs and concentrate. Mix well. Press into the bottom and sides of a 9-inch nonstick pie pan.

Bake for 5 minutes. Cool before filling. If using a no-bake filling, chill and serve; otherwise, bake as directed.

Recipe Hint: *This crust gets soggy if it sits for longer than 1 day. It can be baked, cooled, and filled another day. You can use other sweeteners: Try orange juice concentrate with peach or apricot pies. Pure maple syrup also works well.*

Healthy Muffins

*Servings: makes
18 muffins
Preparation Time:
15 minutes
Cooking Time:
35 minutes*

1½ cups hot water or apple juice
1 cup applesauce
½ cup honey
½ cup raisins
1 cup unbleached white flour
1 cup whole wheat flour

1 cup oat bran
2 cups oatmeal
1½ teaspoons baking soda
1 teaspoon cinnamon
½ teaspoon pumpkin pie
    spice

Preheat the oven to 350 degrees.

Mix the hot water, applesauce, honey, and raisins together and let rest for 10 minutes.

Combine all the dry ingredients in a large bowl and mix well. Add the wet ingredients to the dry and mix. Do not overbeat. Pour into a nonstick muffin pan and bake for 35 minutes. Let rest in the muffin pan for 5 minutes after removing from the oven to make them easier to remove from the muffin pan.

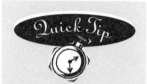

Quick Tip

Cooking breads and muffins in nonstick pans will make removal much easier, but sometimes they still tend to stick. If you let them cool they will pull away from the sides of the pan and pop right out.

Egg Substitute

*Servings: variable
Preparation Time:
2 minutes
Cooking Time:
5 minutes*

¼ cup flaxseed meal   ¾ cup water

Place the ingredients in a small saucepan and slowly bring to a boil. Cook, stirring constantly, for 3 minutes. Store in a covered jar in the refrigerator. Use 1 tablespoon of mixture to replace each egg.

Recipe Hint: This works very well for binding, such as in burgers and loaves. It also works well for cookies, quick breads, and cakes. The consistency of the mixture should be like raw egg whites.

Prune Puree

1 12-ounce package pitted
   prunes

¼ cup light corn syrup
¾ cup water

Servings: variable
Preparation Time:
   5 minutes

Combine the prunes and corn syrup in a food processor and process briefly. Slowly add the water while processing and process until very smooth. Store in a covered jar in the refrigerator.

Recipe Hint: *Use this puree to replace the fat in recipes: Use half the amount the original recipe calls for. Be sure to choose prunes that are not preserved in sulfur dioxide—many people have an allergic reaction to this substance. This is an acceptable substitute for Wonderslim Fat & Egg Replacer, Just Like Shortenin', or Lekvar Filling.*

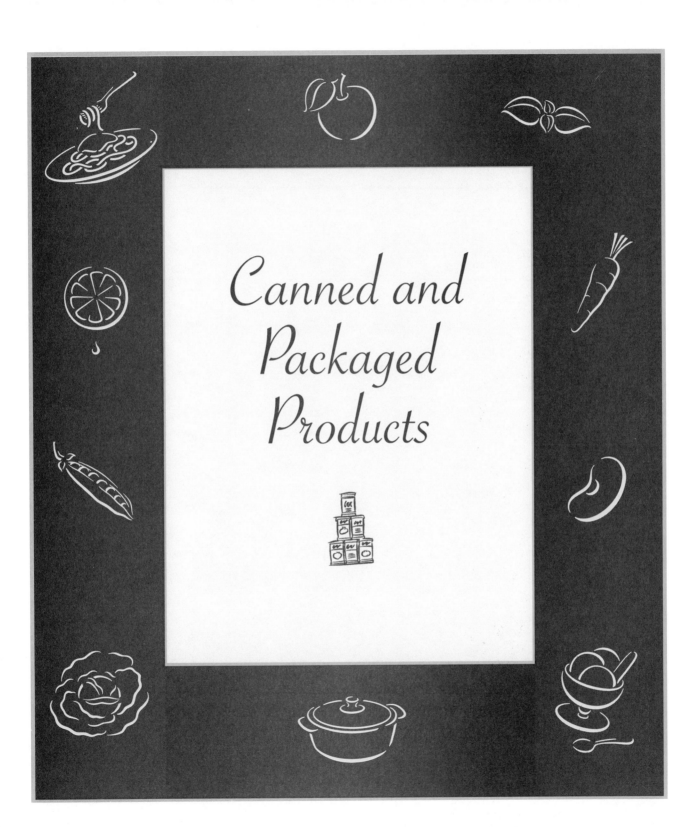

Canned and Packaged Products

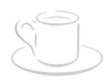

The foods in this section contain no animal products. The foods in the basic list are low in fat (there are no oils added to the ingredients) and simple sugars. These foods are processed as little as possible, but they often contain salt and other additives. People sensitive to these ingredients may need to avoid some of these products. Please read the labels.

The Richer Foods section contains products high in simple sugars and fat. The High–Simple Sugar Foods section contains foods with concentrated simple sugars, such as barbecue sauces, jellies, jams, and nonalcoholic wines. There are lots of calories in these foods and the simple sugars will raise cholesterol and triglyceride levels in sensitive people.

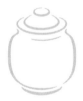

The High-Fat Foods section contains animal product substitutes, such as soy cheeses, soy yogurts, burger mixes, and milks. They are made from high-fat soy products and nuts, and a few may contain added oils. They are often highly processed. They are better for you than the alternative made from animal products, but they are rich, high-fat foods that should be eaten sparingly by healthy people and not at all by those trying to lose weight and regain lost health.

CANNED AND PACKAGED PRODUCTS

Cold Cereals

Alvarado St. Bakery: Organic Granola

Arrowhead Mills: Wheat Flakes, Bran Flakes, Oat Bran Flakes, Corn Flakes, Puffed Wheat, Puffed Rice, Puffed Millet, Puffed Corn, Nature O's, Amaranth Flakes, Spelt Flakes, Kamut, Multi-grain Flakes

Barbara's Bakery: Corn Flakes, Breakfast O's, Brown Rice Crisps, Shredded Wheat, Shredded Spoonfuls, High 5, Frosted Funnies, Startoons Frosted Honey Crunch, Startoons Frosted Cocoa Crunch, Raisin Bran, Breakfast Biscuits

Breadshop's: Health Nuggets, Low Fat Cereal with Organic Grains, Cinnamon Grins, Krinklie Grains, Krispie Corn Flakes, Low Fat Cinnamon Raisin, Low Fat Raisin Cereal, Multi-Grains Grins, Shapes 'N Honey

Health Valley: Honey Clusters and Flakes: Apple Cinnamon, Honey Crunch; Organic Bran Cereal with Raisins, 100% Natural Bran Cereal with Apples and Cinnamon, Real Oat Bran Cereal-Almond Flavored Crunch, Organic Healthy Fiber Multi-Grain Flakes, Organic Blue Corn Flakes, Organic Oat Bran Flakes with Raisins, Organic Fiber 7 Flakes, Organic Amaranth Flakes, Organic Oat Bran Flakes, Organic Raisin Bran Flakes, Fat-Free Golden Corn Fruit Lites Cereal, Oat Bran O's, Stone Wheat Flakes, Fat-Free Granola

Kellogg Co.:   Nutri-Grain: Corn, Wheat, Nuggets, etc.

Kolln: Oat Bran Crunch

Nabisco: Shredded Wheat

Nature's Path Food: Manna: Millet Rice Flakes, Multi-Grain Flakes; Fiber O's, Corn Flakes, Heritage O's, Heritage, Multi-grain, Millet Rice

Perky Foods: Crispy Brown Rice, Nutty Rice

Post: Grape-Nuts

Trader Joe's: Fat Free Granola-Apple Strawberry

U.S. Mills: Erewhon: Wheat Flakes, Kamut Flakes, Aztec, Super-O's, Corn Flakes, Raisin Grahams, Honey Crisp Corn, Galaxy Grahams, Apple Strudels, Banana O's; Skinner's Raisin Bran, Skinner's Low Sodium Raisin Bran, Uncle Sam Cereal

Weetabix Co.:   Grainfields: Wheat Flakes, Corn Flakes, Raisin Bran, Wheetabix Whole Wheat Cereal

Hot Cereals

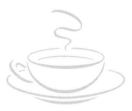

American Cereal Corp.:   Country Choice: Old Fashioned Oats, Apples 'N Cinnamon, Quick Oats, Maple Syrup, and Regular

Arrowhead Mills: Instant Oatmeal: Maple Apple Spice, Original Plain; Bear Mush, Cracked Wheat, 7 Grain, Oat Bran

Barbara's Bakery: 14 Grains

Dr. McDougall's Right Foods: Oatmeal & 4 Grains with Real Maple Sugar, Oatmeal & Wheat with Real Apples & Cinnamon

Fantastic Foods: Wheat 'N' Berry Oatmeal, Cranberry Oatmeal, Banana Nut

Golden Temple Bakery: Oat Bran

Kashi Company: Kashi (some sesame seeds)

Lundberg Family Farms: Hot 'n' Creamy Rice Cereals: Cinnamon Raisin, Amber Grain

Maple Leaf Mills: Red River Cereal: Original, Creamy Wheat, and Bran

Mercantile Food Co.:   American Prairie Organic Hot Cereals

Pritikin Systems: Hearty Hot Cereal: Apple Raisin Spice

Quaker Oats Co.:   Quaker Oats, Quick Quaker Oats

Stone-Buhr Milling: Hot Apple Granola, 7-Grain Cereal

Stone Ground Mills, Inc.:   7-Grain Cereal, Cracked Wheat Cereal, Hot Apple Granola, Scotch Oats, Old Fashioned Rolled Oats

U.S. Mills: Skinner's Oat Bran, Skinner's Toasted Oat Rings; Erewhon: Barley Plus, Brown Rice Cream, Oat Bran with Toasted Wheat Germ, Apple Cinnamon Oatmeal, Apple Raisin Oatmeal, Maple Spice Oatmeal, Dates and Walnuts Oatmeal, Oatmeal with Added Oatbran

Acceptable Milk Substitutes

American Natural Snacks: Harmony Farms: Fat-Free Rice Drink

Eden Foods: Eden Rice Beverage, Edensoy Vanilla Soy Milk

Equinox: Equi-Milk

Grainaissance: Amazake Rice Drink, Amazake Light

Health Valley Foods: Soy Moo (low-fat), Fat-Free Soy Moo

Pacific Foods of Oregon: Pacific Lite

Sovex Natural Foods: Better Than Milk Light
Vitasoy U.S.A.:   Vitasoy Light-Original 1%
Westbrae Natural Foods: Non Fat West Soy Milk, West Soy Lite (1% fat) Plain
White Wave: Silk (1% Fat)

Hot Drinks

Adamba Imports Int.:   Inka
Bioforce of America: Coffree, Bambu
Bolt's Old World Grain Co.:   Gaia's Café
California Natural Products: Dacopa
Eden Foods: Yannoh
General Foods Corp.:   Postum
Libby, McNeil, & Libby: Pero
(many manufacturers):   Herbal teas
Mapi: Raja's Cup
Modern Products: Sipp
Richter Bros.:   Cafix
Sundance Roasting Co.:   Sundance Barley Brew
Teeccino Café: Original, Almond Amaretto, Chocolate Mint, Vanilla Nut
Worthington Foods: Kaffree Roma

Soy Sauces

Edward & Sons Trading Co.:   Ginger Tamari
Kikkoman Foods: Kikkoman Lite Soy Sauce
Live Food Products: Bragg Liquid Aminos
San-J International: Tamari Wheat Free Soy Sauce
Westbrae Natural Foods: Mild Soy Sauce

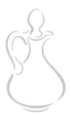

Salad Dressings

American Health Products: El Molino Herbal Secrets
Ayla's Organics: Oil Free: many varieties
Cook's Classics: Cook's Classics Oil Free Dressings: Italian Gusto, Country French, Garlic Gusto, Dijon, Dill
Hain Pure Foods: Fat Free Salad Dressing Mix: Italian, Herb
H.J. Heinz Co.:   Weight Watchers Dressing: Tomato Vinaigrette, French

Kozlowski Farms: Fat Free Dressings: Zesty Herb, Honey Mustard, South of the Border, Raspberry Poppy Seed

Kraft: Oil Free Italian (high salt)

Nakano USA: Seasoned Rice Vinegar

Nature's Harvest: Oil-Free Vinaigrette, Oil-Free Herbal Splendor

Pritikin Systems: No Oil Dressing: Ranch, Tomato, Italian, Russian, Creamy Italian, etc.

Rising Sun Farms, Inc.: Oil Free Salad Vinaigrettes and Marinades: Raspberry Balsamic, Garlic Lovers, Dill with Lemon, Honey & Mustard

S & W Fine Foods: Vintage Lites Oil-Free Dressing

St. Mary Glacier: St. Mary's Oil Free Salad Dressings: many flavors

Sweet Adelaide Enterprises: Paula's No-Oil Dressing: Toasted Onion, Roasted Garlic, Garden Tomato, Lime & Cilantro, Lemon Dill

The Mayhaw Tree: Vidalia Onion Vinegar

Trader Joe's: No Oil Dill & Garlic Dressing, Italian

Tres Classique: Grand Garlic, Tomato & Herb French Dressing

Uncle Grant's Foods: Uncle Grant's Salute-Honey Mustard Tarragon Dressing

W.M. Reily & Co.: Herb Magic: Vinaigrette, Italian, Gypsy, Zesty Tomato, Creamy Cucumber

Other Sauces

Annie Chun's Gourmet Foods: Fat Free Mushroom Sauce, Oil Free Teriyaki Sauce

Ayla's Organics: Cajun, Curry, Szechwan, Thai Sauce

Baumer Foods: Crystal Hot Sauce

B.F. Trappey's Sons: Red Devil Louisiana Hot Sauce

Durkee-French Foods: Red Hot Sauce

Edward & Sons Trading Co.: Stir Crazy Vegetarian Worcestershire Sauce

Gourmet Foods: Cajun Sunshine

J. Sosnick & Son: Kosher Horseradish

Lang Naturals, Inc.: Fat Free Sauces: Honey Mustard, Ginger, Tangy Bang! Hot Sauce, Garlic Steak Sauce, Thai Peanut Sauce (richer), Ginger Stir-Fry Sauce, Honey Mustard Sauce, Sweet & Sour Sauce, Indian Curry Sauce

Lea & Perrins: Lea & Perrins Steak Sauce, HP Steak Sauce

Nabisco Brands: A1 Steak Sauce
New Morning: Corn Relish
Oak Hill Farms: Vidalia Onion Steak Sauce, Three Pepper Lemon Hot Sauce
Organic Food Products, Inc.:   Parrot Brand Enchilada Sauce
Organic Gourmet: Miso Paste: Honey, Apple
Reese Finer Foods: Prepared Horseradish, Old English Tavern Sauce
Renfro Foods, Inc.:   Sauces & Relishes
St. Giles Foods Ltd.:   Matured Worcestershire Sauce

Seasoning Mixtures

Alberto-Culver Co.:   Mrs. Dash: Low Pepper-No Garlic, Extra Spicy, Original Blend, etc.
Barth's Nutrafoods: NutraSoup: Vegetable
Bernard Jensen Products: Broth or Seasoning Special Vegetable Mix
Estee Corp.:   Seasoning Sense: Mexican, Italian
Hain Pure Food Co.:   Chili Seasoning Mix
Maine Coast Sea Vegetables: Sea Seasonings: Dulse with Garlic, Nori with Ginger, etc.
Modern Products: Vegit-All Purpose Seasoning, Onion Magic, Natural Seasoning, Herbal Bouquet, Garlic Magic
Parsley Patch: All Purpose, Mexican Blend

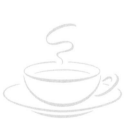

Soups—Dry Packaged

Dr. McDougall's Right Foods: Baked Ramen Noodles-Chicken Flavor, Baked Ramen Noodles, Beef Flavor, Pasta with Beans Mediterranean Style, Rice & Pasta Pilaf Chicken Flavor, Minestrone & Pasta Soup, Split Pea with Barley Soup, Tortilla Soup with Baked Tortilla Chips, Pinto Beans & Rice Southwestern Style, Tamale Pie with Baked Chips
Eden Foods: Ramen: Buckwheat, Whole Wheat
Fantastic Foods: Rice & Beans, Five Bean Soup, Cha-Cha Chili, Vegetable, Barley, Couscous with Lentils, Country Lentil, Black Bean Salsa Couscous, Pinto Beans and Rice Mexicana; Ramen Noodles: Chicken-Free, Tomato, Vegetable Curry, Miso

Health Valley Foods: Pasta Italiano, Fat-Free Cup of Soup-Marinara, Garden Split Pea with Carrots, Spicy Black Bean with Couscous, Zesty Black Bean with Rice, Chicken Flavored Noodles with Vegetables, Lentil with Couscous

Nile Spice Foods: Lentil Soup, Black Bean Soup, Split Pea Soup, Chili 'n' Beans; Pack It Meals: Black Bean, Red Beans and Rice, Lentil Curry

Pacific Foods of Oregon: Chef's Classics: Caribbean Black Beans and Rice, Savory Lentil, Minestrone, Cajun Red Beans & Rice, Curried Lentils & Rice

Sahara Natural Foods: Casbah: Hearty Harvest, Original Couscous, Jambalaya, Morrocan Stew, La Fiesta

Sokensha Co.:   Soken Ramen

The Spice Hunter: Moroccan Couscous, Mediterranean Minestrone, Cantonese Noodle Soup, French Country Lentil, Kasba Curry, Kasba Curry with Rice Bran, Mandarin Noodle Soup

Trader Joe's: Ramen Soup, Brown Rice Ramen, Soba Noodles

U.S. Mills: Erewhon Japanese Misos: Genmai Miso, Kome Miso, Hatcho Miso, Mugi Miso

Westbrae Natural Foods: Ramen: Whole Wheat, Onion, Curry, Carrot, Miso, Seaweed, 5-Spice, Spinach, Mushroom, Buckwheat, Savory Szechwan, Oriental Vegetable, Golden Chinese; Instant Miso Soup: Mellow White, Hearty Red; Noodles Anytime-Country Style

Wil-Pak Foods: Taste Adventure Foods: Black Bean, Curry Lentil, Split Pea, Red Bean, Navy Bean, Minestrone, Red Bean Chili, Black Bean Chili, Lentil Chili, 5 Bean Chili

W.M. Reily & Co.:   Bean Cuisine Soup

Soups—Canned

Fair Exchange, Inc.:   Shari's Bistro Soups: Tomato with Roasted Garlic, Great Plains Split Pea, Indian Black Beans and Rice, Spicy French Green Lentil, Mexican Bean Burrito Soup/Dip

Hain Pure Food Co.:   Fat-Free Soup: Vegetarian Split Pea, Vegetarian Veggie Broth

Health Valley Foods: Organic Potato Leek Soup, Organic Mushroom Barley Soup, Organic Black Bean Soup, Organic Split Pea Soup, Organic Minestrone Soup, Organic Lentil Soup; Fat-Free Soups: 14 Garden Vegetable Soup, Vegetable Barley, Country; Corn & Vegetable, 5 Bean Vegetable, Vegetable Soup-Tomato Vegetable, Split

Pea & Carrots, Lentil & Carrots, Black Bean & Vegetable; Fat-Free Carotene Soups: Italian Plus, Super Broccoli, Vegetable Power; Organic Soups: Mushroom Barley, Potato Leek, Tomato, Black Bean, Split Pea, Minestrone, Vegetable
Little Bear Organic: Bearitos Fat-Free Soups
Mercantile Food Co.:   American Prairie Vegetable Bean Soup
Muir Glen: Organic Tomato Soup
Pritikin Systems, Inc.:   Vegetable Broth, Vegetarian Vegetable
Real Fresh: Andersen's Split Pea Soup
Trader Joe's: Mostly Unsplit Pea Soup, Bean and Vegetable Duet Soup, Tomato Vegetable Soup, Swabian Rice and Vegetable Soup
Westbrae Natural Foods: Fat Free Soups of the World: Great Plains Savory Bean, Santa Fe Vegetable, Louisiana Bean Stew, Alabama Black Bean Gumbo, Old World Split Pea, Spicy Southwest Vegetable, Rich Mediterranean Lentil

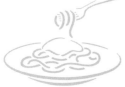

Dry Packaged Grains and Pastas

Arrowhead Mills: Wholegrain Teff, Wheat-Free Oatbran Muffin Mix, Griddle Lite Pancake & Baking Mix; Quick Brown Rice: Spanish Style, Vegetable Herb, Wild Rice and Herbs
Aurora Import & Dist.:   Polenta
Berhanu International Ltd.:   Authentic Olde World-Lentils Divine
Continental Mills: ala-cracked wheat bulgur
Fantastic Foods: Rice: Brown Basmati Rice, Plain, Brown Jasmine; Couscous, Whole-Wheat Couscous; Quick Pilaf: Savory Couscous, Brown Rice with Miso, Spanish Brown Rice, Three Grain with Herbs
J.A. Sharwood & Co.:   Sharwood's India Pilau Rice
Jerusalem Natural Foods: Jerusalem Tab-ooleh
Liberty Imports: Instant Polenta
Lundberg Family Farms: One-Step Entrees: Chili, Curry, Basil; Rizcous, Quick Spanish Fiesta Pilaf, Quick Brown Rice
Melting Pot Foods: Po River Valley Risotto; Marakesh Express: Couscous, Wild Mushroom, Lentil Curry
Near East Food Prod.:   Spanish Rice, Wheat Pilaf, Taboule, Lentil Pilaf Mix
Nile Spice Foods: Whole Wheat Couscous, Couscous Salad Mix, Rozdali
Pritikin Systems: Mexican Dinner Mix, Brown Rice Pilaf

Quinoa Corp.:   Quinoa
Sahara Natural Foods: Casbah Timeless Pilafs: Couscous, Lentil, Spanish, Bulgur, Wheat
San Gennaro Foods, Inc.:   Polenta
Sorrenti Family Farms: Rising Star Ranch: Fiesta Rice, Harvest Rice, Pasta Roma
Texmati Rice: Basmati Brown Rice
The Food Merchants: Kamut Pasta Pilaf Southwestern Blend
Tipak: Couscous, Couscous Express, Polenta Express
Trader Joe's: Sante Fe Rice, Creole Rice, Spanish Rice
Wil-Pak Foods: Taste Adventure: Black Bean Flakes, Pinto Bean Flakes
W. M. Reily & Co.:   Pasta & Beans

Bean and Vegetable Dishes (Frozen or Refrigerated)

Bird's Eye, General Foods: Country Style Rice (microwave)
California & Washington Co. (C&W):   Just Thaw Salad (Sweet Corn and Black Bean), Pepper Strips; Vegetable Stand Combinations: many varieties
Cascadian Farm, Inc.:   Three Rice Medley, Wild Tiger Stirfry
Trader Joe's: Spicy Bean Medley
United Foods: Pictsweet Express; Microwavable Vegetables

Frozen Potatoes

Bel-air: Hash Browns
Cascadian Farm: Organic Country Style Potatoes
California & Washington Co. (C&W):   Whole Red Potatoes
J.R. Simplot Co.:   Okray's Hash Brown Potato Patties
Mr. Dell Foods: Hash Browns
Ore-Ida Foods: Hash Browns, Potatoes O'Brien
Pacific Valley Foods: French Fry Style Potatoes (fat-free)
Sno Pac Foods Inc.:   Potatoes O'Brien

Canned and Bottled Beans and Vegetables

Beatrice/Hunt-Wesson: Rosarita No Fat Refried Beans
Brazos Products: Cajun Bean Dip
Bush Bros. & Co.:   Bush's Deluxe Vegetarian Beans

Del Monte:　Dennison's Chili Beans in Chili Gravy

Eden Foods:　Great Northern Beans, Pinto Beans, Adzuki Beans (all glass jars)

Garden of Eatin', Inc.:　Fat Free Bean Dips; Baja Black Bean, Smoky Chipotle

Goya Foods:　Black Beans

Greene's Farm:　Diced Carrots, Cut Green Beans, Garden Corn, Garden Peas, Refried Beans, Baked Beans

Guiltless Gourmet:　Bean Dips (bottled)

Hain Pure Food Co.:　Fat Free Bean Dips, Fat Free Vegetarian Refried Beans (black and pinto), Spicy Vegetarian Homestyle Chili

Health Valley Foods:　Fast Menu Vegetarian Cuisine: Western Black Bean & Veggies, Hearty Lentils & Vegetables; Tofu Vegetarian Cuisine: Baked Beans with Tofu Wieners, Lentils with Tofu Wieners, Black Beans with Tofu Wieners; Boston Baked Beans, Spicy Vegetarian Chili with Beans-no salt, Mild Vegetarian Chili with Lentils, Mild Vegetarian Chili with Lentils-no salt; Fat-Free Chili: Mild Black Bean, Spicy Black Bean, 3 Bean

H.J. Heinz:　Vegetarian Beans in Tomato Sauce

Little Bear Organic Foods:　Bearitos Beans & Rice: Cuban Style, Cajun Style; Mexican Style Bearitos Bean Dip (black or pinto); Bearitos Fat Free Refried Beans, Bearitos Fat Free Baked Beans; Bearitos Chili: Spicy, Orig., Black Bean

Mercantile Food Co.:　Canned Beans: Kidney, Navy, Black, etc.

Progresso Quality Foods Co.:　Cannellini Beans, Black Beans

Santa Cruz Fine Foods:　Fat Free Bean Dips, Fat Free Guacamole Dip, Black Bean & Corn Salsa

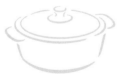

S & W Fine Foods:　Honey Mustard Baked Beans, Maple Sugar Baked Beans, Pinquitos, White Beans, Chili Beans with Chipotle Peppers, Maple Syrup Beans, Deli-Style Bean Salad, Mixed Bean Salad, Dill Garden Salad, Succotash, Garden Style Pasta Salad, Chili Makin's

Stop & Shop Supermarket Co.:　Chick Peas

Trader Joe's:　Kidney Bean Chili, Black Bean Chili, Fat Free Pinto Bean Dips, Fat Free Black Bean Dips, Pineapple Salsa, Raspberry Salsa

Walnut Acres:　Garbanzo Beans, Pinto Beans

Westbrae Natural Foods:　Organic Canned Beans

Whole Earth:　Baked Beans

Salsa

Edible Ecstasies, Inc.:   Sonoma Salsa: Original, Verde, Chili Ajo
Emerald Valley Kitchen: Salsa, Green Salsa
Garden of Eatin':   Great Garlic, Hot Habanero Fiery Salsa, Cha Cha Corn Salsa, Smoky Chipotle
Guiltless Gourmet: Picante Sauce
Hain Pure Food Co.:   Salsa
La Victoria Foods: Chili Dip, Salsa Jalapẽno, etc.
Muir Glen: Salsa
Nabisco Brands: Ortega Green Chile Salsa
Native Foods: Fire Roasted Red Salsa
Nature's Harvest: Salsa
Organic Food Products, Inc.:   Salsa, Smoked Garlic Salsa
   Garden Valley Naturals: Chunky Salsa, Roasted Garlic Tomato, Sun Dried Tomato, Chunky Black Bean; Parrot Brand: Salsa, Tomatillo Salsa
Pace Foods: Picante Sauce
Pet: Old El Paso Salsa
Pritikin Systems: Salsa
Santa Barbara Olive Co.:   Chunky Olive Salsa
Spectrum Naturals, Inc.:   Aylas Organics: Salsa
Trader Joe's: Salsa Authentica, Salsa Verde
Tree of Life: Salsa
Tribal Sun Foods: Authentic Fiesta Salsa
Ventre Packing Co.:   Enrico's Salsa

Spaghetti Sauces

Beatrice/Hunt-Wesson: Healthy Choice Spaghetti Sauce
Campbell Soup Co.:   Healthy Request Marinara Sauce
H.J. Heinz Co.:   Weight Watchers Spaghetti Sauce with Mushrooms
Muir Glen: Organic Pasta Sauces: Cabernet Marinara, Sun Dried Tomato, Garlic and Onion, Italian Herb, Sweet Pepper and Onion, Tomato and Basil
Nature's Harvest: Rocket Pesto
Organic Food Products, Inc.:   Millina's Finest Fat-Free Pasta Sauces: Basil, Zesty Basil, Hot'N'Spicy, Tomato and Mushroom, Tomato and Basil Marinara with Fresh Herbs, Marinara with Zinfandel, Sweet Pepper and Onion, Smoked Garlic, Garden Valley

Naturals: Sun Dried Tomato, Garden Vegetable, Tomato Mushroom, Zesty Tomato Basil, Roasted Garlic

Pritikin Systems: Spaghetti Sauce (Original, Chunky Garden Style)

Pure & Simple: Johnson's Spaghetti Sauce

Robbie's: Robbie's Fat-Free Spaghetti Sauce

Sierra Quality Foods: Muir Glen Fat-Free Pasta Sauce

Sonoma Gourmet: Tomato Caper Herb Sauce

S & W Fine Foods: Simply Wonderful California Pasta Sauces

Trader Joe's: Fat-Free Organic Spaghetti Sauce, Trader Giotto's Italian Garden Fresh Vegetable Spaghetti Sauce

Tree of Life: Fat-Free Pasta Sauce

Ventre Packing Co.: Enrico's Fat-Free Pasta Sauce

Westbrae Natural Foods: Ci'Bella Pasta Sauce (no salt, no oil)

Canned Tomato Products

American Home Foods: Ro-tel Diced Tomatoes and Green Chilies

Beatrice/Hunt-Wesson: No Salt Added Tomato Paste, No Salt Added Tomato Sauce, No Salt Added Stewed Tomatoes, No Salt Added Whole Tomatoes

Contadina Foods: Tomato Puree, Tomato Paste

Del Monte: Tomato Sauce, Tomato Paste, Diced Tomatoes, Chunky Tomatoes; Stewed Tomatoes: Cajun Recipe, Mexican Recipe, Italian Recipe, and Original Style Stewed Tomatoes with Onions, Celery, Green Peppers

Eden Foods: Crushed Tomatoes

Health Valley Foods: Tomato Sauce

Ital Trade, USA: Pomi: Strained Tomatoes, Chopped Tomatoes

Organic Food Products, Inc.: Millina's Finest: Original Fancy California Tomato Paste, Diced Tomatoes (in juice), Stewed Tomatoes, Whole Tomatoes (peeled)

Progresso Quality Foods: Tomato Paste, Tomato Puree

Sierra Quality Canners: Muir Glen Organic Tomato Products

S & W Fine Foods: Ready-Cut Peeled Tomatoes; Tomato Sauce: Thick & Chunky; Stewed Tomatoes: Cajun Recipe, Mexican Recipe, Italian Recipe

Trader Joe's: Tomato Sauce

Walnut Acres: Tomato Puree, Tomatoes

Breads

Alvarado Street Bakery: Oil-Free Breads and Buns

Breads for Life: Sprouted 7-Grain Bread, Sprouted Wheat with Raisin, Sprouted Rye Bread

Brother Juniper's Bakery: Oil Free Breads: Cajun Three Pepper, Oreganato, Whole Wheat

Burns & Ricker: Crispini

Cedarlane Foods: Fat Free Whole Wheat Tortillas, Whole Wheat Lavish Bread

Dallas Gourmet Bakery: Kabuli Pizza Crust

Food for Life: Sprouted Grain Breads

French Meadow Bakery: French Meadow Brown Rice Bread

Garden of Eatin':   Bible Bread-reg. and salt free, Thin-Thin Bread, Swedish Rye, Pita Puffs

Grainaissance: Mochi: Plain, Raisin, Cinnamon, Mugwort, Organic

Great Harvest Bread Co.:   Great Harvest Bakery: Honey Wheat, 9-Grain, Rye Onion Dill, Country Whole Wheat

Health Valley Foods: Fat Free Muffins

International Baking Co.:   Mr. Pita

Interstate Brands: Pritikin Bread: Rye, Whole Wheat, Multi-Grain

Lifestream Natural Foods: Essene Bread

Nature's Hilights, Inc.:   Brown Rice Pizza Crust

Nature's Path Foods: Manna Bread

New England Foods Co.:   Whole Wheat Milldam Pouch Bread

Nokomis Farms: Country Loaf-Sourdough

Norganic Foods Co.:   Katenbrot (Rye Bread)

Oasis Breads: Creative Crust Dinner Shells

Pure Grain Bakery: Pumpernickel, Gourmet Rye, and more

Ryvita: Crisp Breads

Snack Cracks: Pizza Crust-Organic Brown Rice

Trader Joe's: Force Primeval Bars (raisin walnut apple bars)

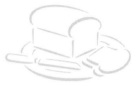

Pastas

Amway Corp.:   Microwave Pasta Ribbons

A. Zerega's Sons: Antoine's Pasta

Bertagni: Gnocchi di Palate

Best Foods, CPC Int.:   Muellers: Twist, Spaghetti, Linguine

Borden: Creamette: Spaghetti, Fettuccine, Shells

China Bowl Trading Co.:   Chinese Noodles, Cellophane Noodles

DeBole's Nutritional Foods:　Curly Lasagna, Elbows, Spaghetti, Corn Pasta (wheat free)

Eden Foods:　Soba (buckwheat), Japanese Rice Pasta, Eden Vegetable Pastas, Udon (Japanese Noodles)

Ferrara Foods:　Gnocchi with Potato

Food for Life Baking Co.:　Wheat-Free Rice Elbows

Garden Time Foods:　Pasta: Spaghetti, Linguine, Rigatoni, Ribbons, Spirals, Bow ties, Trumpets, Corkscrews

Golden Grain Macaroni Co.:　Spaghetti, Macaroni, Rotini, Lasagna, Manicotti

Health Foods:　MI-del: Spaghetti, Macaroni, Alphabet

Health Valley Foods:　Spaghetti Pasta; Spinach, Whole Wheat, Amaranth, etc.

International Delicacies:　Antonio Deniro; Rigatoni, Fusilli, etc.

JSL Foods, Inc.:　Amber Farms Spinach Pasta Wraps

Mrs. Leepers, Inc.:　Michelle's Natural 2 Minute Pasta: Vegetable, Medley, Angel Hair; Mrs. Leepers Pasta: Organic Vegetable, Organic Whole Wheat, Organic Kamut, Rice Pasta, Corn Pasta; Eddie's Organic Pasta: Spaghetti, Rotelli, Corkscrews, Bow ties, Trumpets, etc.

Nanka Seimen Co.:　Chow Mein Udon

Pastariso Products:　Brown Rice Pasta (wheat free)

Purity Foods, Inc.:　Vita Spelt Pasta

Quinoa Corp.:　Quinoa Spaghetti (wheat free)

Reese Finer Foods:　Da Vinci Pasta: Orzo, Spaghetti, Alphabet, etc.

Ronzoni Foods Corp:　Radiatore-79, Linguine, Fusilli, Rotelle, Spaghetti

Sokensha Co.:　Soken Jinenjo Noodles

The Food Merchants Inc.:　Spaghetti, Elbows, Rotelle, Orzo

Tutterri's:　Pasta

U.S. Mills:　Erewhon Japanese Pastas: 40% Buckwheat Soba, 80% Buckwheat Soba, Udon, Ramen Pasta, Ramen with Dashsi

Westbrae Natural Foods:　Spaghetti Pasta: Spinach, Whole Wheat; Lasagna Noodles: Spinach, Whole Wheat; Whole Wheat Somen, Udon, Soba

Burger Mixes and Meat Substitutes

Arrowhead Mills: Seitan Quick Mix
Boca Burger Co.:   No Fat Meatless Boca Burger
Fantastic Foods: Nature's Burger: Barbecue Flavor, Fantastic Falafel
Fearn Natural Foods: Breakfast Patty Mix
Garden of Eatin', Inc.:   Vegetable Jerky: Western Roast, Hot & Spicy BBQ, Pepperoni Pardner
Knox Mountain Farm: Wheatballs, Chick'n Wheat, Not-So-Sausage
Lightlife Foods, Inc.:   Smartdogs, Lightburgers, Smart Deli Thin Slices, Savory Seitan, Meatless Gimme Lean!
Sahara Natural Foods: Casbah Perfect Burger
Sante Fe Organics: Hickory Smoked Seitan and others
Sweet Earth Natural Foods: Seitan
The Pillsbury Co.:   Green Giant: Harvest Burgers for Recipes
Turtle Island Foods: Superburgers
Vegetarian Health Society: Vegetarian Hamburger Bits, Vegetarian Beef Chunks
White Wave, Inc.:   Veggie Burgers: Prime Burger, Seitan: Traditional; Seasoned Seitan, Veg. Philly Steak Slices, Vegetarian Fajita Strips
Wildwood Natural Foods: Fat Free Wild Dogs
Worthington Foods: Better N' Burgers, Granburger, Natural Touch Fat Free Vegan Burger, Ground Meatless
Yves Veggie Cuisine: Deli Slices, Veggie Pepperoni, Canadian Veggie Bacon, Veggie Wieners, Chili Dog, Original Bagel Dog, Chili Bagel Dog

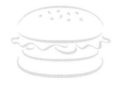

Pretzels

Anderson Bakery Co.:   Oat Bran Pretzels
Barbara's Bakery: Organic Whole Wheat Pretzels: Honey Sweet, 9 Grain, Mini
Frito-Lay, Inc.:   Baked Rold Gold Pretzels
Granny Goose Foods: Stick Pretzels 100% Natural Bavarian Pretzels-salted, unsalted
J & J Snack Foods: Super Pretzels (frozen)
Laura Scudder's: Mini-Twist Pretzels, Pretzel Sticks, Bavarian Pretzels
Little Bear Organic Foods: Organic Mini-Twist Pretzels
Newman's Own Organics: Bavarian Fat Free Pretzels

Snyder's of Hanover: Sourdough Hard Pretzels-salted, unsalted
Wege Pretzel Co.:   Hard Pretzels

Crackers

Auburn Farms Inc.:   Fat Free 7 Grainers, Spicy 7 Grainers (except pizza), Fat Free Spud Bakes (original only)
Baja Bakery: Rice & Bean Tortilla Bites
Barbara's Bakery: Crackle Snax, Lightbread
Burns & Ricker: Fat Free Party Mix, Fat Free Bagel Crisps
Edward & Sons Trading Co.:   Baked Brown Rice Snaps
Lifestream Natural Foods: Wheat & Rye Crispbread
Little Bear Organics: Bearitos Baked Harvest Snackers: Caramel, Orig.
Nabisco Foods, Inc.:   Snack Wells Cracked Pepper Crackers
O. Kavli A/S: Kavli Norwegian Crispbread
Pacific Grain: No Fries: Plain Potato, Tortilla Snacks
Parco Foods: (Hol-Grain) Brown Rice Lite Snack Thins, Whole Wheat Lite Snack Thins
Quaker Oats Co.:   Qrunch 'Ums Cinnamon Cookie Puffs
Ralston Purina Co.:   Natural Ry-Crisp
R.W. Frookies, Inc.:   Fat Free Crackers: Frisps
Sandoz Nutrition Corp.:   Wasa Crispbread: Lite Rye, Hearty Rye
San-J International: Brown Rice Crackers
Shaffer, Clarke & Co.:   Finn Crisp
Snack Cracks: Organic Rice Crackers: Tamari, Lightly Salted
Soken Products: Sesame Wheels: Brown Rice
Stella D'Oro Biscuit Co.:   Fat Free Bread Sticks
Trader Joe's: Fat Free Garlic & Herb Crackers
Tree of Life: Fat-Free Saltines; Fat-Free Crackers: Corn and Salsa, Toasted Onion, Garlic and Herb, Cracked Pepper
Venus Wafers, Inc.:   Fat Free Crackers: Garden Vegetable, Toasted Onion
Westbrae Natural Foods: Brown Rice Wafers

Rice Cakes

Glenn Foods: Brown Rice Treat
H.J. Heinz Co.:   Chico San: Millet Buckwheat, and more
Hollywood Health Foods: Mini Rice Cakes: Apple Cinnamon, Teriyaki

Koyo Foods, Inc.:   Rice Cakes: Millet, Dulse, Hijike, Buckwheat, Plain, Mixed Grain

Lundberg Family Farms: Rice Cakes: Wild Rice, Wehani, Brown Rice, Premium Sesame, Premium Rye with Caraway, Buckwheat, Mochi Sweet; Brown Rice Chewies, Brown Rice Crunchies, Organic Brown Rice, Organic Salted Popcorn, Organic Unsalted Popcorn, Mini Rice Cakes

Pacific Rice Products: Mini Crispys: Apple Spice, Raisin 'N' Spice, Italian Spice, Natural Sodium Free

Quaker Oats Co.:   Rice Cakes (lightly salted), Corn Cakes, Caramel Corn Cakes

The Hain Food Group: Mini Rice Cakes: Plain, Apple Cinnamon; Mini Munchies Fat-Free: Chocolate Mint Crunch, Peach Cobbler, Banana Split

Trader Joe's: Mini Rice Cakes: Plain, Caramel Corn

Tree of Life, Inc.:   Bite Size Snack Fat-Free Rice Cakes: Apple, Cinnamon, Plain

Westbrae Natural Foods: Teriyaki Rice Cakes

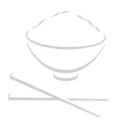

Chips

American Specialty Foods: Smart Temptations Tortilla Chips

Barbara's Bakery: Basically Baked Organic Tortilla Chips, Amazing Bakes Tortilla Chips

El Galindo Mexican Foods: Oil-Free Salted Baked Tortilla Chips, Oil-Free Blue Corn Baked Tortilla Chips

Frito-Lay, Inc.:   Baked Tostitos (Salted and No Salt only)

Garden of Eatin':   California Bakes Tortilla Chips

Good Health Natural Foods, Inc.:   Fat-Free Good Health Baked Potato Sticks

Guiltless Gourmet: No Oil Tortilla Chips: White Corn, Original, No Salt, Chili and Lime

H.J. Heinz Co.:   Weight Watchers Apple Chips

Little Bear Organic Foods: Baked Tortilla Chips

Mexi-Snax Inc.:   Bake-itos Baked Tortilla Chips: Regular, Pico de Gallo, Blue Corn

R.W. Garcia Co.:   Oven Baked Blue Corn Tortilla Chips

Santa Cruz Chips Co.:   Baked Multigrain Tortilla Chips, Baked Organic Blue Corn Tortilla Chips

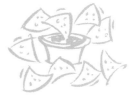

Synergy Systems Corp.:   Childers Natural Potato Chips

Taco Works Inc.:   Eva's Fat Free Potato Chips
Trader Joe's: Baked Tortilla Chips

Popcorn

Arrowhead Mills: Popcorn
Country Grown Foods: Gourmet Popcorn
Energy Food Factory: Poprice
Glacial Ridge Foods: Country Grown-Gourmet Popcorn
H.J. Heinz Co.:   Weight Watchers Microwave Popcorn
Home and Garden: Yellow Popcorn
Lapidus Popcorn Co.:   Lite-Corn
Little Bear Organic Foods: Organic Microwave Popcorn
Nature's Best: Nature's Cuisine (natural popcorn)
Specialty Grain Co.:   Pop-Lite Microwave Popcorn

Baking Ingredients

Eden Foods: Kuzu Root Starch, Agar Agar
Ener-G Foods: Egg Replacer
Fruitsource: Fruitsource Sweetener
Natural Food Technologies, Inc.: Wonderslim Fat & Egg Replacer, Wonderslim Low-Fat Cocoa Powder
Sandoz Nutrition: Featherweight Baking Powder
Sokol & Co.:   Solo Lekvar Prune Plum Filling
Sucanat North America Corp.:   Sucanat
Sunsweet Growers: Lighter Bake
The Plumlife Company: Just Like Shortenin'
The Rumford Co.:   Rumford Baking Powder

RICHER FOODS

HIGH–SIMPLE SUGAR FOODS

Canned Fruit Products

California Custom: Orchard Naturals Fruit
Del Monte: Fruit Naturals: Diced Peaches, Mixed Fruit
Dole Packaged Foods Co.:   Pineapple Chunks (in unsweetened juice), Crushed Pineapple (in unsweetened juice), Pineapple Slices (in unsweetened juice)
Leroux Creek Foods: Fruit Sauces
S & W Fine Foods: Nutradiet: Sliced Peaches, Grapefruit, Apricot Halves, Pear Halves, Sliced Peaches, Peach Halves; Mandarin Oranges (natural style in its own juice), Grapefruit (natural style in its own juice)
The Valley Growers: Libby's Lite: Sliced Peaches, Pear Halves

Barbecue Sauces and Ketchup

Beatrice/Hunt-Wesson: Hunt's All Natural Thick & Rich Barbecue Sauce, No Salt Added Tomato Ketchup
Health Valley Foods: Catch-Up Tomato Table Sauce
Kingsford Products: K.C. Masterpiece Original Sauce
Lang Naturals, Inc.:   Honey Barbecue Sauce
Mrs. Renfro's: Mrs. Renfro's Barbecue Sauce
Pure & Simple: Johnson's Ketchup
Ridg's Finer Foods: Bull's Eye Original Barbecue Sauce; Robbie's Sauce: Barbecue Sauce-mild and hot, Sweet & Sour, Hawaiian Style, Ketchup
The Mayhaw Tree: Barbecue Sauce
Tim's Gourmet Foods: Tim's Barbecue Sauce
Ventre Packing Co.:   Enrico's Catsup
Westbrae Natural Foods: Fruit Sweetened Catsup, UN sweetened Un-Catsup; Fat Free Barbecue Sauce: Orig., Zesty

Jellies, Jams, and Syrups

Anderson's: Pure Maple Syrup
Camp: Pure Maple Syrup

Clearbrook Farms: Fruit Spreads
Deller Foods, Inc.:   MacLean & Larochelle Fruit Spreads & Syrups, Just Honey & Fruity Spreads
Eden Foods: Barley Malt
Knudsen & Sons: All Fruit Fancy Fruit Spreads: Concord Grape, Blueberry, Cranberry, etc.; Syrups: Raspberry, Boysenberry, Fruit N' Maple, Blueberry, Strawberry
Kozlowski Farms: Apple Chutney, Fruit Jams
Lundberg Family Farms: Sweet Dreams Brown Rice Syrup
Maple Creek Farms: Pure Maple Syrup
M. Polaner: All Fruit (jams)
Nature's Harvest: Kiwi Preserve
Rising Sun Farms: Sugar Free Preserves
Robertson Food International: Pure Fruit Conserve
Shady Maple Farms: Maple Syrup
Honey by many manufacturers
Sorrell Ridge Farm: Sorrell Ridge Fruit Only: Apricot, Grape, etc.
Spring Tree Corp.:   Pure Maple Syrup
The J.M. Smucker Co.:   Smucker's Simply Fruit: Red Raspberry, Strawberry, Blueberry, etc.
Timber Crest Farms: Dried Tomato Chutney
Westbrae Natural Foods: Brown Rice Syrup

Breakfast Bars

Barbara's Bakery: Barbara's Nature's Choice Fat Free Fruit Filled Cereal Bars: Apple Filled, Blueberry Filled, Strawberry Filled, Raspberry Filled, Peach Filled and Cranberry Filled; Nature's Choice Fat Free Granola Bars: Multigrain, Apple Apricot, Apple Blueberry, Apple Raspberry
Health Valley: Fat Free Apple Bakes, Fat Free Raisin Bakes, Fat Free Date Bakes; Fat Free Fruit Bars: Apple, Date, Apricot, Raisin; Crisp Rice Bars: Apple Raisin Cinnamon; Fat Free Granola Bars: Raspberry, Blueberry, Date Almond, Strawberry, Raisin; Fat Free Healthy Tarts
Nature's Warehouse: Start Wells Breakfast Bars: Oatmeal Date, Berry
Trader Joe's: Fat Free Bars

Cookies

Auburn Farms, Inc.:   Fat-Free Jammers, Brownies
Health Valley Foods: Fat-Free Apple Spice Cookies, Fat-Free Raisin Oatmeal Cookies, Fat-Free Jumbo Fruit Cookies: Apple and Raisin; Fat-Free Delight Cookies: Date and Apricot, Fat-Free Fruit Center Cookies: Raisin Apple, Date, Apricot, Raspberry, Apple; Fat-Free Mini Fruit Center Cookies: Raspberry-Apple, Peach-Apricot, Strawberry
Natures Warehouse: Fat-Free Fig Bars; Fat-Free Cookies: Cherry, Oatmeal, Caramel Crisp, Banana
R.W. Frookies, Inc.:   Fat-Free Cookies, Obies Cookie Jar: Chewy Oatmeal Raisin Cookie Mix, French Vanilla Cookie Mix

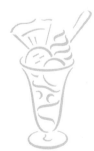

Puddings

Dr. McDougall's Right Foods: Rice Pudding with Real Vanilla & Cinnamon
Grainaissance: Amazake Pudding: Lemon
Hain Pure Foods: Super Fruits Dessert Mix
Lundberg Farms: Elegant Rice Pudding: Cinnamon Raisin
New Market Foods, Inc.:   Cook and Serve Pudding: Vanilla, Brown Rice, Butterscotch
Tree of Life: Island Tapioca-Small Pearl, Large Pearl, Granulated

Ice Desserts

Ben & Jerry's: Fat Free Sorbet
Cascadian Farm: Sorbet
Dole Packaged Foods Co.:   Fruit Sorbet, Fruit N' Juice Bars, Dole Sun Tops-Real Fruit Juice Bars
Ferraro's: Natural Juice Sticks
Frozfruit Corp.:   Frozfruit: Strawberry, Raspberry, Lemon, Cantaloupe, Lime, Orange, Cherry, Pineapple
Garden of Eatin':   Frozen Joy: Watermelon, Mango, Cantaloupe, Lemon-Lime, Strawberry; Fruit Glacé: Passion Fruit, Lemon, Raspberry, Pineapple
Haagen-Dazs Co., Inc.:   Sorbet
Howler Products: Rainforest Fruit Sorbets
J & J Snack Foods Corp.:   Luigi's Real Italian Ice

Nouvelle Ice Cream Corp.:   This is Bliss
Real Fruit Co.:   Real Fruit Chunky Sorbet
R.W. Frookies, Inc.:   Cool Fruits Fruit Juice Freezers
The J.M. Smucker Co.:   Fruitage Premium Frozen Dessert-Raspberry
Turtle Mountain, Inc.:   Sweet Nothings

Nonalcoholic Wine

Ariel Vineyards: Premium Wines Without Alcohol: Chardonnay,
    Cabernet Sauvignon, Blanc, Rouge, White Zinfandel, Riesling,
    Sparkling Wines

HIGH-FAT FOODS

Milks

Devansoy Farms, Inc.:   Solait Instant Soy Beverage
Eden Foods: Eden Blend, Endsoy (other than vanilla)
Ener-G Foods: Pure Soyquick
Health Valley Foods: Soy Moo
Imagine Foods: Rice Dream
Mitoku Co. Ltd.:   Supersoy
Pacific Foods of Oregon: Organic Soy Beverage
Westbrae Natural Foods: Westsoy Plus
Wholesome & Hearty: Almond Mylk, White Almond Beverage

Burger Mixes and Meat Substitutes

Fantastic Foods: Nature's Sausage
Ivy Foods: Wheat Meat: Sun Burgers, Grilled Burgers, Hearty Origi-
    nal, Chicken Style, Sausage Style, Beyond Roast Beef, Beyond
    Chicken Patties, Beyond Turkey
Lifestream Natural: Vegi-Patties
Lightlife Foods, Inc.:   Wonderdogs
Mudpie Frozen Foods: Veggie Burgers
Sweet Earth Natural Foods: Veggie Burgers: Fiesta Rice, Savory
    Soy, Seitan
White Wave, Inc.:   Veggie Life Burger, Vegetarian Sloppy Joe,

Sandwich Slices, Snack'n Savory Tofu, Baked Tofu, Tofu Steaks, Teriyaki Tempeh Burger, Tempeh Burger

Wholesome & Hearty: Garden Veggie, Garden Vegan

Burger Mixes with Tofu

Fantastic Foods: Tofu Burger Mix, Tofu Scrambler Mix
Sahara Natural Foods: Gyros Greek Classics
Sovex Natural Foods: Better Than Burger?, Really Chili
Sunfield Foods: Lite Chef Country Barbecue

Dairy Substitutes

Northern Soy, Inc.:   Soy Boy Ravioli
Sharon's Finest: Vegan Rella
Soyco Foods: Soymage Sour Cream Style Soy Cheese: Soymage-Cheddar Style, Mozzarella Style, Jalapeño Style, Grated Parmesan, Soy Single
Soyen Natural: Soya Latte (nondairy yogurt)
White Wave: Dairyless Yogurt

Desserts

Imagine Foods: Dream Pudding
Tofutti Brands: Better Than Yogurt, Lite Lite Tofutti

Contributions

With our warmest appreciation we would like to thank the following people for their contributions to this book:

John and Bonnie Bogenberger of Sun Valley, CA—Pasta with Chili Sauce

Joyce Bowen of Santa Rosa, CA—Creamy Vege Soup and Tri-Bean Barbecue

Mary Bresson of Livingston, TX—Bresson's Noodles and Beans

Louise Burk of Santa Rosa, CA—Jicama Matchsticks

Laurie J. Cain of San Diego, CA—Southwestern Bean Salad

Barbara Coberly of Los Angeles, CA—Radish Salsa

Jayne DeLawter of Sebastopol, CA—Basmati Rice Salad and Spicy Bulgur with Vegetables

Jack Dixon of Santa Rosa, CA—Almost Instant Breakfast and Jack's Breakfast Sandwich

Linda DuPuy of Plymouth, MI—Beans and Things

Lisa Dylina of Merced, CA—Southwest Brown Rice

Jason Elliot of Santa Rosa, CA—Couscous Salad with Spicy Soy Yogurt Dressing

Harry Forst of Novato, CA—Fat Free Fudge

Ginger Grafues of Santa Clarita, CA—Easy Fruit Tart

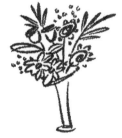

Susan Haskins of Santa Rosa, CA—Artichoke Pasta Sauce

Jean Hines of Chiloquin, OR—Thai Tofu with Cashews

Sharon Hughes of Middletown, CA—Quick Wisconsin Chili

Suzanne Laitner of Rohnert Park, CA—Tofu and Black Bean Stew

Mary Lane of Mission Viejo, CA—Mexican Black Bean Tortilla Soup

Jennifer Luftop of Fort Worth, TX—Cuban Potatoes

Skip and Barbara Marsh of Fresno, CA—Mexican Lasagne

Dollie McAlister of Sebastopol, CA—Sweet Breakfast Rice

Karen Meldrum of Alameda, CA—Cream of Vegetable Soup and Rice Pudding

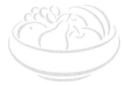

Kit Miller of Danville, CA—Fast Pasta and Salsa and Spicy Chili and Chips

Cynthia Murata of Waipahu, HI—Cynthia's Eggplant Spaghetti Sauce and Barbecued Tofu Sauce

Patricia Oberg of Sebastopol, CA—Fat-Free Hummus

Diane Perkins-Davis of Lakeland, FL—Black Bean Pizza and Black Eyed Pea Scramble

Sylvia Polk of Fairfield, CA—Creamy Sun Dried Tomato Sauce

Sandy Rockenbaugh of Marysville, OH—Tex-Mex Lasagne

Suzanne Ross of Orangevale, CA—Broccoli Pasta Soup

Ellen Smith of Cypress, CA—Ellen's Bean Soup

Julie B. Smith of Tarzana, CA—Fiesta Black Bean Dip

Marilyn Strauch of Folsom, CA—California Pasta Salad and Mexi Soup

Anita Sullivan of Eagan, MN—Slow-Cooked Lentil Stew

Ronald Ushijima of La Mirada, CA—Oatmeal Masa Porridge

Linda Williams of Mission Viejo, CA—Williams Crockpot Chili

Ruth Youngsman of Mount Vernon, WA—Tortilla pie crust tip

Index

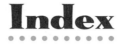